Acknowledgments

My grateful thanks, as ever, to my agent, June Clark, for always keeping my personal and professional best interests at heart; for her spot-on guidance and reality checks; and for her sensitivity in advocating for people with different ways of being.

In compiling this volume, I was aided immeasurably by terrific parents who submitted great questions; my gratitude to those who took time out of their busy lives to send them:

Rummana Ali-Zaman, Kathy Baas, Holly Berlin, Debbie Bradshaw, Traci Cornette, Margaret Deddy, Deborah A. Delp, Marcella Kramer, Marcella Diaz, Kim Goodman, Carol Hammer, Julia Howerin, Stanley P. Jaskiewicz, Trieste Kennedy, Kari Main, Tami Malzahn, Laura Manley, Karin Renard, Kathy Scarfone, Sheryl Shenk, Lesa Shusta, Nancy West, and Tamara Wilson.

Lisa Rudy, a mom and also the online guide for About.com's autism site, deserves special recognition for never hesitating to spread the word about my endeavors to serve the autism community.

Contents

Introduction

At first glance, the title of this book, *The Autism Answer Book*, may seem a bit presumptuous. After all, how can any book propose to be "the" answer book on autism when hundreds of others have already been written on this special needs topic? Although the title is somewhat of a misnomer, *The Autism Answer Book* does endeavor to be a comprehensive reference guide for parents, caregivers, and educators—with a twist. Both the format and my unique qualifications make it an easy-to-use and fairly definitive guide.

Herein, you will find many of the questions most commonly asked by concerned and wondering parents, such as:

- Will my child ever recover from autism?
- What exactly caused my child to have autism?
- How can I get my child to use the toilet?
- How do I explain my child's autism to relatives and extended family?
- How do I deal with my other children's envious feelings because of the extra attention I give my child with autism?
- Should I give my child medication for her autism?
- What's causing my child's public meltdowns?
- My spouse has similar traits as my child—is my spouse autistic too?

Dozens more questions—submitted by *real* parents—will be answered gently and compassionately but from a unique, "inside-out" perspective. That is, this handbook is the first question-and-answer primer in which autism, in all its mystery and beauty, is decoded, deconstructed, and respectfully explained by someone who, for the most part, has been through it. As an individual with Asperger's syndrome, my position as your author and guide differs from that of other experts. It is my intent to support your understanding of autism in the same way as your child might if he could sit you down and walk you through it every step of the way. Besides, who better to describe what it's like *and* put to rest unfair myths and stereotypes?

You'll also discover three very significant themes embedded throughout the text of *The Autism Answer Book*, themes which are generally absent in more clinically oriented books: the presumption of intellect, the technique of prevention instead of intervention, and the strategy of fostering self-advocacy in your child. Grasping these most fundamental and salient of autistic tenets will go a long way toward strengthening your relationship with physicians, educators, therapists, siblings, and relations, and, of course, your child with autism. Many opportunities to enrich and understand these bonds await you on the path toward a bright and hopeful future. So, let's begin!

Chapter 1 WHAT IS AUTISM?

- ■ What is autism exactly?
- ■ What are the classic characteristics of autism?
- ■ Is having autism like having Parkinson's or Alzheimer's?
- ■ Who "discovered" autism?
- ■ I've heard autism referred to as a "spectrum disorder." What does that mean?
- ■ What is PDD-NOS?
- ■ What is Rett's disorder?
- ■ What is childhood disintegrative disorder?
- ■ What is Asperger's syndrome?
- ■ What is the difference between high-functioning autism and Asperger's syndrome?
- ■ Why am I reading and hearing so much about autism these days?
- ■ What causes autism?
- ■ Are certain people more at risk for getting autism than others?
- ■ Can autism be screened or determined with prenatal testing?
- ■ Are children born with, or do they acquire, autism?
- ■ Is my child's autism my fault?
- ■ What are some early warning signs that a parent should look for?
- ■ Does having autism mean my child is mentally retarded or intellectually impaired?
- ■ What does it mean to "presume intellect" in my child?
- ■ Does having autism mean my child has a precocious savant skill, like *Rainman*?
- ■ Will my child's autism get worse with age?
- ■ What is the cure for autism?
- ■ If there's controversy about a cure, should I still have hope for my child?
- ■ Who is best equipped to help raise my child?
- ■ What kind of medication do I give my child for autism?
- ■ What can I do to help my child with autism to grow and learn like other kids?
- ■ Will my child always need care and supervision?

What is autism exactly?

The word *autism* is derived from the Greek word *autos*, or "self," as in *autonomous*. It has been used to describe individuals who appear to be self-contained or who exist in their own little world, an inner realm seemingly set apart from others. These individuals have been clinically characterized as intentionally withdrawn and lacking in social reciprocity due to their communication difficulties or seeming disregard for social norms, as demonstrated through repetitive actions such as repeated hand flapping or infinitely spinning the wheel of a toy truck instead of rolling the truck along on all four tires.

From a physiological perspective, autism is a common neurological anomaly that may preclude the body from properly receiving signals transmitted by the brain, resulting in misfires and disconnects. Thus, people with autism may be unable to speak (or to speak reliably), to move as they would wish, or carry themselves with grace and complete agility. You've experienced autistic-like symptoms if you've ever transposed or stuttered your words unintentionally, or if you've awakened in the middle of the night to discover your arm is "asleep" from the elbow down and cannot be willed by your brain to move of its own accord.

Autism is a unique and different way of being, a natural variation of the human experience. Those who are autistic are often inherently gentle and exquisitely sensitive. They may perceive the world through a multifaceted prism more complicated and interesting than the view of those who are considered "typical." The autistic experience brings many gifts to appreciate and challenges to master—as will be discussed—as one attempts to assimilate with the world at large.

What are the classic characteristics of autism?

Your child *may* be exhibiting symptoms of autism if he:

- Seems challenged in communicating through the use of nonverbal communications such as making eye contact or using appropriate facial expressions, body language, and gestures.
- Seems to have difficulty developing friendships with children his own age.
- Doesn't seem to enjoy showing you what he's doing, bringing something he likes to you, or pointing out things he finds interesting.
- Seems to prefer to play alone, or will allow others to play only if they are helpful in abetting a "master plan" he's devised.
- Experiences a delay in talking or doesn't develop speech.
- Talks, but seems to find it difficult to begin a conversation or keep a conversation going in ways that would be considered socially appropriate.
- Uses language in unusual ways, such as referring to himself in the third person or repeating certain words or phrases.
- Doesn't engage in make-believe play or play that imitates social models (such as things mommy or daddy does).
- Has a very strong and intense preoccupation with a certain item or topic.
- Engages in specific rituals or routines, and may become upset if they are disrupted.
- May make physical movements that are out of the ordinary, such as constant rocking, flapping his hands, or spinning his body.

Some of these symptoms may present themselves in ways that might be tempting to label as dysfunctional, but they are really your child's attempts to conjoin with the world. You might typically observe these telltale traits in the areas of social interaction, language usage, and the way your child plays, about or before the time he is three years old. The preceding criteria are not diagnostic, and if you have concerns about your child's development, you should follow up with your pediatrician.

Is having autism like having Parkinson's or Alzheimer's?

At present, autism is not associated with other neurological disorders such as Parkinson's or Alzheimer's, but correlations can be made in the ways autism may manifest similarly (the classic characteristics listed in the preceding question). One significant difference is that autism is not considered a "disease" like these other ailments, and is therefore not degenerative; modern medicine does not yet have the knowledge or expertise to prevent conditions like Parkinson's or Alzheimer's from progressively encumbering those who experience them. It is apt, however, to compare these conditions with autism in that autism involuntarily imposes on one's neurology and hinders speech and movement. Autism's uncommon movement or vocal limitations should not be considered as originating in one's willful volition any more than forgetfulness due to Alzheimer's or trembling due to Parkinson's is willful.

Who "discovered" autism?

In 1801, French physician Jean-Marc Gaspard Itard documented what is regarded as the earliest recorded account of autism in his published work, *The Wild Boy of Aveyron*. Itard became ward to a "feral" twelve-year-old boy, whom he dubbed Victor, a child plucked from his solitary, nude existence in the forest the previous year. It was believed that Victor, who was without speech, was abandoned by his family and subsisted without any form of human contact. Itard's descriptions of Victor's behavior while in his care were later regarded to correlate with classic symptoms of autism.

But the individual credited with first defining autism is Leo Kanner (1894–1981), a Johns Hopkins University School of Medicine child psychiatrist. In his 1943 paper, "Autistic Disturbances of Affective Contact," Kanner presented his collective observations of children who demonstrated traits now associated with classic characteristics of autism. Kanner's findings created a new understanding of children previously misdiagnosed with schizophrenia or mental retardation. His diagnostic criteria were temporarily referred to as Kanner's syndrome, Kanner's psychosis, or Kanner's autism.

Coincidentally, Hans Asperger (1906–1980), an Austrian pediatrician, published similar findings in early 1944, just months after Kanner's publication; both men were unaware of each other's research, and yet, curiously, both men used the word *autistic* to describe their observations (which was originally used to describe the tendency to view life in terms of one's own needs and desires, or someone morbidly self-obsessed). Asperger's work focused on a group of children who appeared to be preoccupied with train timetables, clocks, and other narrow interests, and who experienced difficulty with social interaction such that they were labeled "odd" or "frankly unusual." Though initially termed *autistic psychopathy*, the collection of traits Asperger documented would eventually become known as Asperger's disorder or Asperger's syndrome. (Please note that the terms *psychosis* and *psychopathy* are germane to a specific clinical era, and, to our modern sensibilities, may be perceived as disrespectful.)

It is likely that autism has always been with us, a part of us, in one aspect or another, even though the condition was only identified in the twentieth century.

I've heard autism referred to as a "spectrum disorder." What does that mean?

There are many degrees of manifestation of autism from highly functional to noncommunicative, and the spectrum refers to the range in which a child's autism-related symptoms fall. To understand the phrase *spectrum disorder,* let's set aside the term *disorder* and focus on *spectrum.* Think about the spectrum of light and color, and consider the infinite variations in hue and subtle gradation of shades that are possible. This is what is intended when the autism spectrum is referenced as such. The manifestations of autism are merely natural nuances and subsets of our own anthropology grouped into similar—but not identical—ways of being.

As presently defined by the American Psychiatric Association's *Diagnostic and Statistical Manual of Mental Disorders,* the autism spectrum consists of five such variations collectively called *pervasive developmental disorders*: autistic disorder (or autism), Asperger's disorder (or Asperger's syndrome), Rett's disorder, childhood disintegrative disorder, and pervasive developmental disorder–not otherwise specified. However, we are all more alike than different in our humanity; just as no two of us is reserved from being indistinguishable, the autistic experience is as unique and individual as each individual is unique. Further, within the fields of politics, sports, or entertainment, for example, there exist many gifted and talented individuals who are all contributing their part within their respective "spectrums." And yet we are all united as human beings, each a worthy participant of the space we occupy.

What is PDD-NOS?

PDD-NOS is the acronym for the clinical diagnosis *pervasive developmental disorder–not otherwise specified.* It is a subgroup within the aforementioned diagnostic category of pervasive developmental disorders. (PDD-NOS is often incorrectly referred to as simply PDD for short, which is improper, because PDD is the overarching category for the autism spectrum and *not* a diagnosis.)

PDD-NOS is ascribed as a diagnosis when an individual, usually a child, does not qualify for the full features of autism or one of the other PDD experiences, and yet the individual is autistic-like in what is clinically defined as "marked impairment of social interaction, communication, and/or stereotyped behavior patterns or interests." In other words, the individual just misses meeting the criteria for autism or Asperger's, but still falls somewhere on the autism spectrum because she exhibits some of the symptoms. PDD-NOS may also be used by physicians who are not well versed in making an autism diagnosis or who prefer to maintain a cautious "let's wait and see" holding pattern. Often, as a child with PDD-NOS grows and develops and the diagnosis is revisited, she has matured into one of the other PDD categories. But on occasion, as a child matures, she may blend so well socially that the diagnosis gets dropped altogether.

What is Rett's Disorder?

Rett's disorder or Rett's syndrome (also just "Rett" or RS) is one of the clinical pervasive developmental disorders. Unlike autism, Rett's (first identified in 1966) tends to impact little girls almost exclusively. Sometime in their early development—usually between five months and four years—such children experience a noticeable slowing of head growth as well as a regression of motor skills and capabilities such as caring for one's personal needs or moving with ease. This loss of motor control can also impact the ability to produce speech where previously spoken language was present.

According to their website, the **International Rett Syndrome Association** is "the only organization dedicated to providing families with the latest medical information, aggressively funding the most promising research, offering meaningful support, raising public awareness, and advocating for those living with the neurological disorder called Rett syndrome." For further information, visit www.rettsyndrome.org.

What is childhood disintegrative disorder?

Similar to Rett's, childhood disintegrative disorder (CDD) is also a pervasive developmental disorder, and is considered rare. With CDD, a child may progress through typical developmental milestones and appear as ordinary as any of his peers. But after the first two years of life, the child may regress inexplicably and lose many previously acquired skills such as toileting, self-care, and the ability to communicate in ways that are understood. The child may also face challenges in developing normal social interactions with other children.

CDD may also be called disintegrative psychosis or Heller's syndrome. Be mindful that while the medical profession is cut and dried about creating such labels, the intent is not personal nor blatantly disrespectful, but simply linguistically clinical. Regardless, such labels can be devastating to any parent who is distraught and confused by their child's unexpected transformation.

What is Asperger's syndrome?

Asperger's syndrome or Asperger's disorder (also just "Asperger") is another pervasive developmental disorder or autism spectrum experience. As mentioned previously, it was first defined by Hans Asperger in the early 1940s. The difference between Asperger's syndrome and autism is that the Asperger's individual develops typically in childhood without any apparent cognitive or developmental delays. In fact, it is not unusual that some children not yet identified as having Asperger's may be diagnosed with hyperlexia, a precocious ability to read and pronounce language beyond what would be usual in someone so young (however, it doesn't mean the child is using the complex language with intent or understanding). Thus, Asperger's can go unnoticed altogether.

Asperger's syndrome is also noted by difficulties understanding how people "work" socially; cultural idioms (sarcasm, double entendre, innuendo) and humor may require explanation before it is clear. Such individuals may become deeply absorbed in topics of special interest or passion, and might excel to the degree of brilliance or giftedness. Others may not feel physically adept or coordinated, or may appear monotone and emotionless.

Speculation is that up to 80 percent of people with Asperger's are self-diagnosed. This may be attributed to the fact that it has only been officially recognized since 1994, or it could be that, for most of their lives, so many pass for "normal" that others simply think them eccentric, peculiar, or hermit-like. Persons of renown reputed to have Asperger's include Ludwig van Beethoven, Emily Dickinson, Henry Ford, Mark Twain, Alfred Hitchcock, *Peanuts* creator Charles Schulz, and Microsoft magnate Bill Gates.

What is the difference between high-functioning autism and Asperger's syndrome?

The term *high-functioning autism* (HFA) is not a diagnosis officially recognized as one of the five pervasive developmental disorders, although it is a quasi-diagnostic label used and often interchanged with that of Asperger's by some prescribing physicians. However, despite some disagreement, it is generally conceded that this is a misapplication of HFA, which may be distinguished by an initial language delay not seen in Asperger's.

Note also that a reverse contention is employed to describe individuals defined as "severely autistic"—that is, *low-functioning autism*. In lieu of semantics, however, of greatest importance is that we place value on the person and not on her label; and no one wants to be described as "low functioning."

Why am I hearing and reading so much about autism these days?

Autism, as an experience and topic of international interest, has been gaining slow momentum since its reclassification in the 1994 publication of the American Psychiatric Association's *Diagnostic and Statistical Manual of Mental Disorders* (DSM). The DSM is *the* mental health clinician's reference tome, consulted by psychiatrists, psychologists, general practitioners, diagnosticians, and other professionals.

With the reclassification, children who may have been diagnosed as having mental retardation or a learning disability became properly identified within the autism spectrum. The prevalence of autism now surpasses other high-profile conditions such as childhood cancer, cerebral palsy, cystic fibrosis, and juvenile diabetes—lending to accumulating scientific and media attention in recent years. Recent statistics released by the federal Centers for Disease Control and Prevention (CDC) cite that 1 in every 166 children is autistic, or nearly 500,000 individuals under age twenty-one—and that doesn't begin to capture the number of adults impacted, for which there is no formal accounting. A 2007 revision of statistics by the CDC indicates that 1 in every 150 children of about eight years of age is now autistic. It is unknown if the rise in statistics is due to proper diagnosis or genetic, social, or environmental factors (read on for more about this).

What causes autism?

That is the question of all questions where this topic is concerned! At present, there is no one source to which any parent, professional, researcher, or scientist can attribute the cause of autism. Theories abound, however, and the most compelling point to genetic suscepti-bility (there's a 3 to 8 percent chance of having a *second* child with autism, and a 30 percent greater likelihood that identical twins will be autistic than fraternal twins) and environmental triggers such as viruses or a reaction to the now-banned mercury preservative, thimerosal, in the mumps-measles-rubella (MMR) childhood vaccine.

Other theories include children's overexposure to television, fathers who were middle aged at conception, and pregnant mothers' exposure to toxic pollutants. A weakened or compromised immune system has also been thought to blame.

Perhaps most significant to acknowledge is not the cause of autism but what autism causes: a call to action by parents and the medical community to understand and address—even embrace—autism in more comprehensive and meaningful ways than they have in the past.

Are certain people more at risk for getting autism than others?

For reasons unknown, autism is four to five times more common in males than females. This prevalency does not, however, constitute having an at-risk status, because autism occurs naturally without regard for race, geographic locale, lifestyle, or socioeconomic status.

Can autism be screened or determined with prenatal testing?

Currently, there is no prenatal test or screening for autism. Interestingly, during summer 2006, a controversy arose in the United Kingdom over a University College Medical School (London) proce-dure to screen for male-gender embryos in families thought to be genetically predisposed to autism. The sex-selection technique would allow families to abort male fetuses and retain female fetuses, because males are more likely to be autistic than females.

Announcement of the university's plans incited strong opposition from advocacy organizations protesting the potential for "designer babies" and the establishment of a society in which only perfection is valued.

Are children born with, or do they acquire, autism?

No one can say with certainty. It is believed that, most often, children are born autistic. Because each child is unique, and autism is a spectrum experience, when and how autism is detected may vary greatly. It may come through in ways that are clear and profound, or subtle and virtually undetectable. Still, a great number of parents assert that their children were not autistic prior to receiving the MMR vaccine, and that after the vaccination—literally overnight—they became autistic. Weaving together both contentions is this: are these children who were born autistic and, as a result of the vaccine trigger, began displaying autistic traits because of their inability to eliminate the mercury in their system—or would they have eventually demonstrated their autism one way or another? David Kirby's bestselling 2005 book, *Evidence of Harm*, investigates the vaccine controversy and its repercussions in depth.

Is my child's autism my fault?

Absolutely not, and let no ill-mannered individual convince you otherwise, despite those who insist on perpetuating the ancient, insulting stereotype that cold, indifferent "refrigerator" mothers are responsible for inducing their children's autism.

What are some early warning signs that a parent should look for?

Indicators that a toddler or young child may be displaying autistic symptoms could include:

- not responding, or appearing not to listen when you speak;
- spending time playing alone;
- echoing others' spoken words, or repeating the same words;
- using gestures to indicate a want, or pulling you to a want instead of using spoken language;
- bouts of intense expressions of frustration (called tantrums by some);
- not wanting to be touched or hugged;
- fleeting or no direct eye contact;
- a need for consistency in schedules and routines;
- fascination with parts of toys instead of the toy itself;
- no apparent understanding of personal safety or danger;
- physical movements (walking or picking things up) that may be inconsistent with typically developing peers;
- acute reactions to sensory sensitivities (sounds, tastes, sensation of fabrics);
- not speaking in two-word phrases by two years old; or
- loss of language or learned skills at any age.

For further information, visit www.firstsigns.org.

Does having autism mean my child is mentally retarded or intellectually impaired?

In a word, no, although popular myth points to the contrary. It has been variously estimated by a number of clinical sources that anywhere from 50 to 90 percent of individuals with autism have mental retardation (excluding individuals with Asperger's). However, this statistic can be misleading, and the linkage of mental retardation and autism is an antiquated stereotype that must be assuaged and relegated to the past.

Because many children with autism do not speak, do not speak reliably, or echo speech, they score 70 percent or below on standardized intelligence quotient tests, which are the clinical criteria for mental retardation. But no one would test in ways that reveal our true intellect if we were without an effective means to communicate, were expected to interact with a stranger in a strange or uncomfortable environment, and were asked to comply with peculiar or misunderstood requests.

The proper response to autism is to re-envision how we conceive it, in the same way we observe the person with cerebral palsy who does not speak reliably and has limbs that cannot be willed into compliance—as with autism, that individual's thought processes are fully intact, and nowhere near as impaired with the same limitations as her physical shell.

When in doubt, *presume intellect* in the person with autism and interact with a belief in his competence as gently and respectfully as you would anyone else.

What does it mean to "presume intellect" in my child?

Presuming intellect requires that you perceive your child's diagnosis in name only, and disregard its label and the myths and stereotypes that may accompany it. It means that—even though your child may not speak, or speak clearly, or appears to be disinterested and not listening—you know fully that he is aware and understands your communications to him. You will need to be especially mindful of demonstrating respect and compassion by not talking about your child in front of him as if it didn't matter, particularly in ways that emphasize his so-called "deficits," or bemoaning the stress your child's diagnosis places on your life, your job, and your marriage and relationships. Presuming intellect necessitates that you partner with your child in collaboration for every aspect of his life, and allow him input and control over the decisions regarding how best to get his wants and needs met—regardless of whether he can talk, has been labeled with autism, or has even been diagnosed with mental retardation. Presuming intellect requires that you look beyond labels to enrich the relationship with your child through a belief that his competence is intact.

Does having autism mean my child has a precocious savant skill, like *Rainman*?

As much as the film *Rainman* illuminated some of the real-life symptoms of autism, it also created a new stereotype: that of the autistic savant. You may, indeed, notice that your child has unique capabilities for remembering dates, statistics, or phone numbers. Your child may intuitively know how to operate electronic appliances and computers without ever looking at an instruction manual. And your child may read well beyond his grade level, or create with an ingenious artistry exceeding that of most adults. On rare occasions, these abilities are truly extraordinary and seemingly without an apparent explanation, such as an affinity for artistic or musical composition.

If this describes your child, it may be tempting to describe such attributes as "gifted," especially if you've felt your child was undervalued by others. But we *all* possess great talents; they define our avocations, vocations, and with whom we relate best.

As much as we must vanquish the myth of autism automatically equaling mental retardation, we must also cease perpetuating the stereotype that persons with autism are savants who should display and perform their advanced skills to our awe and amazement. When we subscribe to this notion, we risk creating a sideshow mentality that emphasizes *what* people are instead of *who* they are. Remember: all human beings are blessed with both gifts and flaws.

Will my child's autism get worse with age?

As noted previously, autism is not a disease or degenerative illness, so it will not advance into deteriorating "stages," so to speak. Your child's autism will not worsen with age, but, as she grows and matures, there will be occasions on which you'll wish to adapt and refine the ways she's learned to navigate people, social situations, and the community in general. Think of it this way: how much French do you remember from high school? Chances are not much beyond a few words and phrases. *But*, if you used French almost every day, you'd be articulate and fluent.

In a similar respect, your child will need to employ helpful behaviors every day of her life in order to attempt to blend. This can feel like using a foreign language to your child: it takes practice, role-playing, and counseling to decipher the "language" of people. It is tricky, confusing, and frustrating to always try to second-guess people, their "secret codes" of communication, and their body language. Your loving support will help your child learn ways of deconstructing human behavior and coping with her frustration. Adults with autism who struggle the most are the ones particularly challenged by these issues, and might be unable to "blend" as seamlessly as others.

What is the cure for autism?

Just as no one knows the cause of autism, the jury's still out on a cure. It is generally conceded that there is no "cure" for autism per se. Adult self-advocates (individuals on the autism spectrum who defend their rights) will explain that autism, and its variations, is a lifelong experience that must be assimilated or sometimes temporarily suppressed in order to integrate with the outside world—though few wish to alter their unique way of being and surrender totally to the status quo. Their motto is, in essence, celebrate not eradicate!

However, there are those parents and professionals who are adamant that they have "recovered" or cured their children through various methodologies (see Chapter 8, Treatment Options, for further details), successfully erasing all traces of autism.

This begs another question: are those children who have been cured no longer autistic, or have they merely learned to manage their autistic traits well enough to pass for "normal"? That is, in striving to extinguish all traces of autism, have parents and professionals caused children to completely suppress autistic urges in favor of compliance, and is that really the same as a cure? The answer lies in eliciting a response from those very children, teenagers, and adults themselves; they are the only persons best able to reply about life with or without the autistic experience.

If there's controversy about a cure, should I still have hope for my child?

Of course! People on the autism spectrum are not incapacitated, and neither is your child—hope abounds. On the journey you are undertaking with your child, you will brave many obstacles along the yellow brick road; but you will also be blessed by encounters with many compassionate and caring individuals who will benefit you in ways you would least likely expect—just when you require their aid most. Always be optimistic and open to the possibilities offered your child by a world that is slowly, but surely, embracing diversity in all its magnificence.

Trust your instincts as a parent. Read, research, and become knowledgeable; talk with other parents about what's worked for them. Good questions to ask when exploring, pursuing, and implementing any program, therapy, or method designed to help your child with autism include the following:

- Is there a way to measure improvement?
- Does the program seem to be helping?
- Is there a specific timeframe in which I should begin to see developmental growth occur?
- Is my child happy, interested, and engaged?
- Is my life less stressful for it?
- Can I replicate what's being offered naturally within the flow of my daily routines?
- Does the program allow my child the opportunity to interact with his peers?

Who is best equipped to help raise my child?

As a parent, you know and love your child best and can best care for your child, although you will certainly benefit from the loving support of family and others. However, generations ago, this would not have been the answer you would have been given. It is important to recognize the history of care for persons with different ways of being; there was a time when parents were urged, if not pressured, to place their children in out-of-home institutional centers in which, parents were informed, their children would be better cared for by professionals trained to support such "handicapped" children. In fact, the term "inmates," usually reserved for those who are incarcerated, was commonly employed to describe institutional charges who lived in such settings.

Hundreds of thousands of parents who made the agonizing choice to part from their children were advised not to have contact with them in many instances, and were told to get on with their lives. They were misled into believing they lacked the wisdom and expertise to love and parent their own children! Add to this the shame and guilt imposed on them because of the stigma of producing a "handicapped" child, and you will understand our egregious past.

Although the concept of institutionalizing children with complex diagnoses has been discarded, there are still occasions on which it is suggested to modern-day parents that their children be "sent somewhere." Do not, under any circumstances, be misled into thinking this holds promise for your child. Segregation is oppression, and the world so dearly needs your child in it to teach empathy, compassion, and tolerance.

This does not mean that specially trained professionals do not have expertise to impart to you and your family, and the value of such will be further discussed.

What kind of medication do I give my child for autism?

Autism is a natural experience. You *do not* medicate a natural experience any more than you'd give medication to someone who is blind because they don't perceive vision with their eyes. Disbelieve anyone who tells you that because your child is autistic, they require prescription medication for "behaviors." Most such medication is offered to quell difficult-to-manage symptoms resulting from hyperactivity, overstimulation, and acute anxiety that, for the most part, could be managed in other ways, as you will learn in the mental health chapter, Chapter 6. All such medication comes with side effects that could be detrimental to your child's very sensitive physiology. This is a real issue for kids who are unable to speak or put language to the adverse effects they're experiencing—that is, if they are even able to make the connection between feeling ill and ingesting new medication. Medication should never be prescribed arbitrarily or for the convenience of sedating someone into compliance, unless an individual presents imminent danger to himself or others. The choice to use medication as one avenue in treatment is a very personal decision on the part of the parent in cooperation with the child's doctor. While there is no medication for autism, as noted, you may choose to medicate adjunct aspects of your child's experience that manifest in mental health diagnoses, if necessary, such as anxiety or depression.

What can I do to help my child with autism to grow and learn like other kids?

Supporting your child to grow and learn as her peers do is a process. As much as we are all more alike than different, the autistic experience comes with its own set of nuances that can hinder the learning process. How successfully your child grows and learns depends on choices that you make *in partnership* with your child wherever possible. It matters not that your child doesn't speak—she is entitled to co-collaborate with you in all matters concerning her life and way of being. She is the only one who knows what helps her learn most effectively.

Trust your intuition: if something doesn't feel "right" no matter how much others insist it's for the best, *don't do it*. Similarly, listen carefully to what your child is telling you—listen not just with your ears *but with your eyes*. Be attuned, attentive, and ever conscious to the myriad manners in which your child communicates.

You will likely be doing a lot of reading, research, and gaining insights from other parents and professionals in the autism field. But remember to temper this information with consideration of the *true* experts—those adult self-advocates with autism who are able to communicate their experience, reflect on their upbringing, and explain their perceived differences in ways no one else can. They represent the voice of the child without a voice, and it is of great importance that we pay them reverence and respect in exchange for their "inside-out" expertise. You may learn more about adults with autism, their lives, and their perspectives through some of the resources offered at the back of this book (many self-advocates are authors).

Will my child always need care and supervision?

The response to this question provides the opportunity to introduce two of the book's main themes (the third being "presume intellect"): the concepts of "prevention instead of intervention" and "fostering self-advocacy." No one can say with certainty what level of care, support, or assistance your child may require into adulthood. As you are raising your child, be mindful of the concept "prevention instead of intervention." In so doing, you'll fast become savvy to always thinking ahead in order to prepare your child for what to expect socially, in educational and vocational environments, and with regard to his sensory sensitivities in new surroundings. And while there will always be unexpected, unanticipated happenings, by teaching your child the concept of prevention instead of intervention, you are imparting the gift of self-advocacy. It's a harsh realization to know that you are ultimately temporary in your child's life; fostering resiliency, independence, and self-reliance to the greatest possible extent will enable your child to be better poised for his future as an adult.

Chapter 2

GETTING A DIAGNOSIS

- How do I know if I should have my child evaluated for autism?
- My child seems to be developing typically but has times when she "zones out" and won't pay attention, but she also doesn't cry or have tantrums as I've read autistic children can do—could she still have autism?
- Where do I start if I suspect something's not right?
- Will my health care insurance pay for my child's evaluation?
- Do I have to travel somewhere special to get my child evaluated?
- What makes a professional qualified to make an autism diagnosis?
- What can I expect of the evaluation process?
- Should I bring anything with me to the evaluation?
- Is there anything I can do to prepare my child for the evaluation?
- My child doesn't talk—will he be given an IQ test?
- How long will it take until I know if my child has autism?
- What if I don't agree with the results of the evaluation?
- What if it's *not* autism?
- If it *is* autism, what now?
- I'm devastated by the autism diagnosis—how do I handle this?
- I feel like I'm being punished with a child who is less than perfect—am I?
- My child was also given *another* diagnosis in addition to autism. Now what?
- Does an autism diagnosis mean I need to think about sending my child somewhere else to live?
- What services are available to my child?
- What will such services cost me?
- I've got to tell someone—who can I talk to?
- Is there anyone I *shouldn't* tell?
- What is "person-first" language?
- Should I tell my child about her diagnosis?
- What is the best way to talk about autism with my child's siblings?
- Some family members don't believe my child's autism diagnosis. How do I handle this?
- Since getting my child's diagnosis, and doing a lot of reading and research, I'm realizing that a lot of the information about the traits of autism is shared by my spouse. Is this possible?
- Will my child ever need to be reevaluated in the future?

How do I know if I should have my child evaluated for autism?

Do not be afraid or hesitant to approach your child's pediatrician if you feel your child is not meeting developmentally appropriate milestones. If you are a first-time parent, your pediatrician can fully inform you as to what to expect developmentally as your child grows and matures.

Do you know other parents of same-aged children against whom you can compare typical child development? Do you have a history of "late bloomers" in your family that didn't walk or talk until a bit beyond what's usual but, ultimately, caught up just fine? Are you perhaps diagnosing your own child because of one autistic symptom in isolation from others (which wouldn't necessarily constitute autism)? Your pediatrician will advise you if your child appears to be experiencing any sort of delay. Parents of children with autism often want to be made aware of their child's diagnosis as early as possible to take advantage of the important developmental toddler years, when children's neurology that affects communication and motor skills is most flexible.

Your pediatrician is not being helpful if he or she is beating around the bush to spare your feelings, withholding information in favor of a "let's wait and see" approach, or isn't experienced in diagnosing autism. Contrast your child's way of being with what you are learning about autism and be prepared to offer specifics if you feel it may apply to your child. When in doubt, seek a second opinion.

My child seems to be developing typically but has times when she "zones out" and won't pay attention, but she also doesn't cry or have tantrums as I've read autistic children can do—could she still have autism?

Be cautious not to rely on autism stereotypes you've come to know through film and television portrayals; they're oftentimes sensational-ized for effect. Also, be certain that you're not overcompensating by applying certain symptoms you've heard or read about to your child.

Sometimes, children who are overly compliant or "too good" (the baby that never cries when put down for a nap) are later diagnosed on the autism spectrum, but don't jump to hasty conclusions. While your child may not qualify for autism criteria, she may qualify for another diagnosis such as sensory integration disorder, attention deficit disorder, or attention deficit/hyperactivity disorder, which is estimated to go undiagnosed 50 percent of the time. Your child's distractibility may correlate to a learning delay, dyslexia, or perhaps a hearing or vision difficulty. Or perhaps it's nothing to be concerned with. Always check your concerns with your child's pediatrician before jumping to conclusions.

Where do I start if I suspect something's not right?

Start by consulting your child's pediatrician. If he or she doesn't feel qualified to diagnosis your child, ask to be referred to another pedia-trician who specializes in developmental concerns; you could be referred to a child psychologist or pediatric psychiatrist or to a specific clinic in a children's hospital or medical center. If you are unaware of professionals who may be helpful other than your child's doctor, consult the Human Services section in the community pages of your local telephone directory. Your county (or neighboring county) should have a Human Services office that houses a wide variety of child, youth, and family professionals. If they aren't able to serve you, they should at least be able to refer you to someone who can. You may also wish to search your library or the Internet for nearby or statewide autism groups that can guide you to helpful, reputable professionals.

In some cases, concerns about your child's development may be brought to your attention by child care or day care providers, because if you work, they may see your child more than you do, and their opinions should be carefully considered. If your child is older, you may be informed by your child's teacher or school psychologist. Your immediate reaction may be to become defensive of your child when approached by someone else, especially if it's done in a confrontational or accusing manner. Remember, the professional caring for your child in your absence may not realize your child's way of being has a name and may, instead, accuse your child of bad behavior or you of poor parenting. Try to set aside any personal inclinations in favor of listening carefully and asking clarifying questions so that you can discern fact from emotional anecdote. This clear-cut information will aid you in following up with professionals who are able to diagnose your child.

Will my health care insurance pay for my child's evaluation?

This may vary depending on what your health care insurance provider covers or what your employer's insurance plan has agreed to. Prior to consulting with a professional who can diagnose your child, check with your insurance provider to ascertain any limitations, restrictions, or special requirements, such as a prescription for services or direct referral from your primary care physician. For diagnostic services such as an evaluation for autism, your health care insurance may cover 100 percent of it or you may be required to pay a deductible or copay.

As far as coverage for additional services, this again will vary depending on your insurer or employer plan. In certain cases, such services are covered but only up to a certain dollar amount or number of sessions, or an insurance rider may be added by the insurer to include traditional therapies such as physical therapy, occupational therapy, or speech therapy. Other insurers will cover no additional therapies. If you suspect your child will require additional professional supports not covered through employer insurance, you may wish to shop for private insurance plans if that's a possibility for you.

If you don't have health care insurance, you'll need to explore other options. Depending on your income level, you may qualify for Medicaid. Your local county system Human Services office can help you determine if you and your family are Medicaid eligible. You may also wish to check out the U.S. Department of Health and Human Services program (www.insurekidsnow.gov) or call 1-877-KIDS-NOW.

Parity laws require that health care insurers must cover physical and mental health services equally. To learn the parity law status in your state, go to the American Academy of Child and Adolescent Psychiatry site at www.aacap.org/legislation/stChart.htm.

Do I have to travel somewhere special to get my child evaluated?

Depending on your location and the availability of qualified professionals who are knowledgeable about autism, you may have to travel to the nearest major metropolitan area or prominent medical center. To do this, you may need to travel to the next county, across the state, or even across state lines. As great an undertaking as this may seem, don't allow yourself to feel daunted or deterred into postponing—this is important stuff, and you and your child will benefit from knowing the truth about her experience as soon as possible. It may take some coordinating with your employer, child care provider, friends or family members to aid you in getting to where you need to be when you need to be there, so plan in advance.

What makes a professional qualified to make an autism diagnosis?

Professionals who should be knowledgeable on the symptoms of autism include developmental pediatricians, pediatric psychologists, pediatric psychiatrists, school psychologists, and other clinicians who are affiliated with children's medical health providers. Such professionals should not only be licensed and certified to practice their profession, they should also be required to maintain a knowledge base current with up-to-date, best-practice information through a set number of annual training hours in a diverse range of pertinent topics relevant to their field (training hours which they are always welcome to exceed). In addition, he or she may further their expertise through participation in clinical studies, consulting with professional peers, authoring books and articles, and reviewing contemporary literature in their respective field through peer-reviewed clinical journals and parenting periodicals.

To learn more about any prospective professional to whom you have been referred, request references or ask for the website of that clinician or his or her employer. Information about his or her education and accreditation, employment history, and awards or achievements for excellence should be noted.

What can I expect of the evaluation process?

Lots of questions! Come prepared to listen carefully to what the doctor is asking and try to answer as directly and concisely as possible. In such a situation, many parents may be understandably filled with lots of nervous anxiety; it may be tempting to want to verbally vent to someone who finally understands your situation and is providing you with validations and assurances. If your child is truly on the autism spectrum, his symptoms and traits will reflect just that; therefore, there's no need to portray your child's behaviors in the worst possible light, nor is there a need to sugarcoat your child's experience—neither approach is helpful. You'll also not be of service to your child if you digress into lengthy storytelling in order to highlight a single challenging incident in great detail, especially in your child's presence.

Respectfully allow the doctor to guide the appointment, and really listen to what he or she is telling you. The doctor should also spend time observing and interacting with your child. Your child may be asked to take an intelligence quotient (IQ) examination, participate in a series of questions or activities as an assessment test, or may be requested to play, possibly in a setting from which he may be observed through two-way glass.

Before the appointment concludes, the doctor should give you the opportunity to ask any additional questions, should give you a sense of when you will receive the evaluation results, and should provide you with his or her contact information if you do not already have it.

Should I bring anything with me to the evaluation?

Bring only what the doctor or his or her nurse practitioner or receptionist has requested that you bring. It will not be helpful if you bring stacks of papers, baby pictures, diaries and journals, homework and artwork, and bulging binders of information if the doctor hasn't asked for it—nor will the doctor have time during the appointment to review it. What you likely will be asked to bring—or sign an advance release of information to access records from your child's primary care physician—will be documentation pertaining to medical, psychological, educational, and family history for your child that will help the doctor determine any delays in typical child development that might indicate autism or another diagnosis. If you have some document that you do not wish to be overlooked, offer to highlight it or otherwise tag it for the doctor's attention.

You may also wish to ask for a copy of the assessment document that will be used in the evaluation (see more about this in the next answer).

Is there anything I can do to prepare my child for the evaluation?

You'll likely be taking your child to a new environment with the expectation that she interact with a stranger while assimilating or taking in unfamiliar sights, sounds, and other sensations. She will be expected to comply with requests that may hold little meaning for her, or that she misunderstands or misinterprets. As stressful as the appointment may be for you, imagine how it is seen through your child's uniquely sensitive lens. This is a situation in which your child may not be at her best—may even succumb to acute anxiety—unless you employ the concept of prevention instead of intervention.

Here are some things you can do in advance of the appointment in order to aid your child in feeling safe, comfortable, and in control:

- Reinforce that the upcoming appointment is with the kind of doctor that only asks questions (as opposed to the kind that pokes and prods and gives shots!).
- Explain the timeframe for the appointment, including starting and ending times, and also wait times.
- Share whatever questions you speculate the doctor may ask your child (try obtaining these in advance from the doctor's nurse practitioner or office staff).
- Show your child the doctor's picture, office, and office location on the Internet. This advance knowledge will empower your child to feel familiar with the doctor.
- Ask that your child help you plot your travel route by obtaining driving directions on the Internet or visually tracing your routes on a map.
- Visit the doctor's office ahead of the appointment day if possible (and explain that it's "just to visit") or ascertain from the office staff information about the environment such as lighting, scents

(which can be really overwhelming in medical environments), noise, and other sensory sensation triggers that may provoke your child.

- Determine typical wait times and whether a more tranquil, alternative environment in which to wait is available if there are delays beyond your appointment time (which, on emergency short notice, may be the bathroom). Try calling ahead before you leave to make certain you're still on schedule.
- Allow your child to take along an object or objects that soothe and fascinate him (such as his length of string, *Star Wars* figure, or plastic straw) to help him quell any anxiety he may be experiencing.
- Formulate with your child questions he'd like to ask the doctor, depending on how or if he communicates.
- Decide just how much or how little you'll share about your child in front of her. Weigh carefully the embarrassment and humiliation your child may feel—and, yes, she really is listening—overhearing you describe her in terms of behaviors, limitations and shortcomings, failures, and defeats.
- Plan a favored activity immediately following the appointment, and keep your promise even if things didn't go as planned.

My child doesn't talk—will he be given an IQ test?

It is likely that some form of intelligence quotient (IQ) examination will be administered in order to determine if your child's level of cognitive functioning (how he thinks and processes information) is on par with that of his peers. Obviously, the child who is absent the ability to communicate verbally is going to be limited by the manner in which the IQ test is given, and a good clinician should be knowledgeable about augmenting an IQ test with other methods of assessment.

In addition to an IQ examination or a variation equivalent, the doctor conducting the evaluation of your child may use other written assessment tools that may involve asking you and your child questions, asking your child to participate in various tasks and activities, or observing how your child plays or interacts with others. If you know your child to have delayed reactions or to require extra process time to act on requests, please ensure that the doctor is aware of this requirement. Assigning your child's diagnosis should result from a combination of tests, observations, and interviews.

How long will it take until I know if my child has autism?

This may vary greatly depending on the doctor's schedule. As a professional clinician, the doctor will require some time to process and absorb his or her observations and findings. You should receive a written summary of the appointment and the doctor's conclusions within 30 days or less. If you haven't heard anything in a timely manner, feel free to call the doctor's receptionist or nurse practitioner to inquire when you might expect to receive the written report.

What if I don't agree with the results of the evaluation?

If you are in disagreement with the results of the evaluation, or if you need clarification about any aspect of it, contact the doctor's office, leave a message, and request that he or she contact you to resolve any issues or concerns you may have. It is important that the evaluation's content is clear to you because it is the document that will aid you in accessing formal and informal services and supports to benefit your child's development. It may be that the evaluation report contains some technical or clinical jargon that simply requires explaining in layperson's terms in order to be understood.

If the doctor has attempted to clarify the evaluation or rationally restates his or her position, and you *still* disagree with it in part or in whole, seek a second opinion.

What if it's *not* autism?

If your suspicions about your child's autism are *not* confirmed by the evaluation report, your child will most likely have been ascribed at least one other diagnosis that may share some similarities with autistic symptoms such as fragile X, sensory integration disorder, attention deficit disorder, or attention deficit/hyperactivity disorder. If, however, you feel strongly that your child has been misdiagnosed, revisit the report's findings with the doctor or nurse practitioner, or seek a second opinion. Be prepared, however, to back up your perspective with evidential information based on your observations. As difficult as it may be to see the forest for the trees sometimes, you *do* know your child best—and you've been his parent far longer than a doctor has spent observing him. If you intend to challenge the diagnosis, be certain you've been thorough in your information gathering in order to make your case for a diagnosis contrary to the doctor's findings.

If it *is* autism, what now?

Congratulations! You've been blessed with an extraordinary child who will be an amazing teacher for you, someone from whom you will learn more about life than in any textbook.

Concurrent with the autism diagnosis, the doctor or nurse practitioner should provide you with literature and contact information for local, statewide, and national supports in the form of service agencies, autism organizations, reading materials, Internet resources, and other professionals who may be of service to you. Take advantage of the materials offered as a starting point as you begin to process and assimilate lots of new information.

I'm devastated by the autism diagnosis—how do I handle this?

Try to pinpoint *why* you're feeling so completely overwrought. Is it because news of the autism diagnosis took you completely off guard, and now you're in mourning, so to speak? You may be feeling numb and deeply upset, grieving the loss of the person you envisioned your child would be, or would become, when she was first born; but this is natural, and will pass in time if you allow yourself to be open to new possibilities.

Are you feeling devastated because whoever broke the news to you painted a gloomy picture of a hopeless future for your child, one of perpetual caregiving and a life absent of many typical achievements? This kind of insensitivity still occurs, and is obviously not helpful if you were given the "bum's rush" as the diagnosis was ascribed, with a parting "do the best you can" or "just take her home and love her" sort of admonishment. Some clinicians who are skilled in what they do lack people skills or are very uncomfortable when breaking surprising news to families.

Your hurt, frustrated, angry, or melancholy feelings may also be compounded by news stories that, more often than not, insist on putting a tragic spin on autism. Rarely do we hear of success stories in the media, so you may be replaying only the most sensationalized portions of what you recall seeing, hearing, or reading about.

Some parents are relieved to know that their child's way of being has a name that can be researched, is not the result of willful misbehavior, and has nothing to do with poor parenting. Many parents believe their greatest resource is being able to connect with another parent in the same situation. The National Parent to Parent Network is one organization that brings together parents in geographic proximity (maybe even in the same town!) who desire to share their stories and experiences; check it out online at www.P2PUSA.org.

Additional supportive resources are listed at the back of this book.

I feel like I'm being punished with a child who is less than perfect—am I?

This question sounds like a longing for spiritual resolve. Studies have shown that families' commitment to their spirituality or religious practices can directly impact their ability to coalesce and overcome obstacles as a family unit. Those families who are devout in their faith have been shown to cope with their children's autism with reduced stress and solid conviction.

One mom who was feeling sorry for herself described her "why me?" mentality as being in "victim mode," until she realized: "why *not* me?" She felt she had been chosen to parent her son because of her humanitarian skills, her ability to advocate loud and clear, and her strength in navigating service systems. Indeed, these traits have served her well in raising her son.

If you persist in feeling persecuted for a prolonged period of time, please consider consulting with someone from a local place of worship or a community counselor in order to sort through the issues and formulate a plan to move forward with optimism.

My child was also given *another* diagnosis in addition to autism. Now what?

As stated previously, you may wish to dispute the doctor's findings if you are in disagreement by providing evidence to the contrary or by seeking another opinion. Although it is not unusual for children with autism to have more than one diagnosis, the legitimacy of a concurrent diagnosis may be questioned or ruled out as your child grows and matures.

It may be that you *are* in agreement with the added diagnoses, and it may even be a relief to understand that your child's symptoms are attributable to other factors. Some diagnoses commonly associated with autism include Down syndrome, mental retardation, fragile X, hyperlexia, obsessive-compulsive disorder, attention deficit disorder, attention deficit/hyperactivity disorder, intermittent explosive disorder, oppositional defiant disorder, sensory integration disorder, anxiety, depression, bipolar disorder, and post-traumatic stress disorder. Each one of these experiences carries its own set of criteria, and will require your knowledge and understanding to learn how any concurrent diagnosis may interface with that of autism.

Does an autism diagnosis mean I need to think about sending my child somewhere else to live?

No! This is outdated thinking. As discussed in Chapter 1, there was an era not so long ago when parents would have been encouraged, instructed, or pressured into placing a child with any uncommon diagnosis into a segregated setting or institution. Today's thinking holds that your child with autism requires the consistency and stability of your unconditional love and support as his parent.

Don't be seduced into thinking that another living arrangement, school, or center can supplant your ability to parent your own child. Remember: you are your child's greatest ally and most ardent advocate, and she needs you to create positive inroads on behalf of her and other children with autism. You will, though, need to ensure that the home environment is one that is generally settled and has structure; your child will likely react adversely to a random home environment that is loud and noisy, chaotic, and filled with overstimulating irritants such as cigarette smoke and strong food odors, or room temperatures that are too high or too low. Be willing and open to making compassionate accommodations to meet the needs of your child in your home.

What services are available to my child?

This may depend on your child's age, which is why you are encouraged to seek a clinical evaluation as early in your child's development as possible. If your child is an infant or toddler, or under the age of five, his autism diagnosis will likely qualify him as eligible for Early Intervention. Early Intervention is a federally mandated program administered by every state to provide services and supports to children with developmental delays who qualify based on an assessment of need.

To learn more about Early Intervention, contact your local county Human Services office, found in the community pages of your telephone directory. Through this office, you may also be able to access other beneficial services and supports for your family, and gain help in doing so from professionals knowledgeable about maneuvering the Human Services system.

According to its website, another federal program, Head Start, "serves the child development needs of preschool children (birth through age five) and their low-income families" by trying to prepare your child for school by kindergarten. The official Head Start website (www.acf.dhhs.gov/programs/hsb) will answer questions you have, help you locate the nearest Head Start office, and guide you to other resources. Ten percent of Head Start enrollments are reserved for children with disabilities, and Head Start is required to fully include those children in programming alongside their peers without disabilities.

Your school district or local university may also be a resource to you through the special education department. Referrals to autism organizations, parent meeting groups, literature, trainings and presentations, and professionals who may support you can result from making these connections.

What will such services cost me?

Early Intervention and Head Start services are available at low or no cost to you, depending on an assessment of your child's needs, income eligibility, and family size. Your health care insurance may also be drawn on to supplement certain therapies and other services.

However, whatever the cost, these programs can definitely be worth it—suggestions, strategies, and techniques offered by professionals whom you will encounter in these programs can help you give your child every advantage to develop her language and motor skills and help her learn how to play with other kids. In addition, you may decide to augment any services your child receives by paying out of pocket for "extras" that might not be deemed as necessary or beneficial by Early Intervention or Head Start professionals, things such as music or art therapy, or animal therapies such as interactions with dolphins or horseback riding.

For older children who qualify, your Human Services agency may aid you in accessing certain therapists or behavioral support staff; your school district may also be a resource in making connections with professionals who can be of service at low or no cost to you.

I've got to tell someone—who can I talk to?

This is a personal decision dependent on your circle of support. Your spouse or co-parent is certainly entitled to know of the diagnosis. But what of immediate family—whose business is it, and whose business will you *choose* to make it?

In desiring to tell someone of your child's autism diagnosis, you surely want reassurances and gentle, loving consolations that everything will be okay. What you don't want is someone whom you thought was a confidant coming back at you with an "I told you so" kind of attitude—someone who will be judgmental and accusatory.

Mentally survey your closest allies. Who can you trust? Who has been there for you unconditionally? Who is the best listener? Who will help you in determining next steps? Who has always thought your child was gorgeous and unique despite his differences? These kinds of questions will guide you in determining with whom you choose to reveal your child's diagnosis.

If you feel alone, and without a trusting ally, do not hesitate to contact the National Parent to Parent Network referenced on page 298, call your local counseling center, or search the Internet for any of the myriad autism websites that offer chat rooms and message boards. In addition to the resources listed at the back of this book, one Internet site with a very active message board for parents supporting other parents is www.autism-pdd.net.

No matter whom you choose to tell about your child's autism diagnosis, you know tears of sadness, joy, and frustration are almost sure to follow. You'll want to kindly and sensitively exercise discretion to ensure you are not emotionally emptying yourself about your child in front of him.

Is there anyone I *shouldn't* tell?

Again, this is a personal decision, but one that should take into account the concept of personal disclosure in respectful consideration of your child—regardless of age. It is not necessary to tell persons with whom you have limited contact or see irregularly. If you don't feel that certain family members would be very supportive, carry on business as usual; you're not obligated to share such private information any more than you would reveal anything similar about yourself of a clinical or medical nature.

What's not helpful is to abide by the popular concept of printing up business-size cards explaining your child's autism in terms of questionable, unusual, or off-the-wall behaviors that you arbitrarily dispense to strangers in the community at the height of your child's public meltdown. Many parents feel they ward off stares and accusations of parental blame by using such cards as "shorthand" to educate onlookers about autism. Although such intentions are pure, they only serve to *reinforce* what those unaware of autism have come to believe in terms of media myths and stereotypes. In other words, by distributing a card about autism to strangers at the mall at the moment your child appears to be tantruming, you are, in essence, conveying, "Yes, this is autism and this is what it looks like." Not only have you "outed" your child in public, you have perpetuated negative precedents that define your child in terms of "behaviors." Instead, practice "prevention instead of intervention" by preparing your child in advance for the different environment or by avoiding the environment altogether.

What is "person-first" language?

Person-first language is a thoughtful demonstration of respect by verbally valuing the individual *before* describing them by their diagnosis or difference. For example, instead of calling someone "an autistic" or saying "autistic child," you would value the person *first* by rightfully stating "child *with* autism." In making the point about person-first language, advocate and mom Kathie Snow asks if you would rather be described as a person with cancer, or as *cancerous?* It is the difference between being sensitive or insensitive, between telling about *who* not *what*.

As you begin to learn about autism, you may understand that persons on the autism spectrum themselves are not particular about person-first language; they may, in fact, refer to one another using slang terms such as *autistics, auties,* and *Aspies.* This does not mean that you should follow suit and abandon using person-first language when communicating with those individuals. Persons on the autism spectrum enjoy a cultural camaraderie that permits them to employ "insider" slang if they choose to, in the same manner that other cultural groups use certain labels in jest or affectionately among themselves but consider it offensive if an "outsider" uses the same terms. Responding respectfully with person-first language compels you to be conscious of your words and aware of how you use them, and that's a good habit to have. You will, in no time, cringe or correct others when you don't hear them using person-first language.

Should I tell my child about her diagnosis?

Honesty is the best policy, and knowledge is power. In fostering self-advocacy, you should initiate an ongoing dialogue with your child about autism as a natural variation on the human experience as soon as you receive the diagnosis. Some adults with autism who were not told from the start or who were misdiagnosed have reported self-loathing and depression for not realizing they were blameless and that their altered way of being had a name. Even if your child doesn't feel different now, she may in the near future and certainly risks being *made* to feel different by her peers.

It's not enough to believe that your child suspects she's different. She is entitled to know that difference has a name and is not her fault—even if you fear "labeling" her. One mom said, "Not telling your child about autism won't make it go away! Wouldn't you tell your child if he has asthma?" Or consider this story: another parent has cerebral palsy but wasn't told until she was a young adult! Instead her parents told her the tremors were all in her head, and she could control her shaking if she wanted to! Disallow this attitude from becoming your child's legacy.

Because many individuals with autism are visual thinkers and learners, you will best be able to communicate autism information through pictures and words tailored to your child's age level. A quick Internet book search will direct you to any number of current titles written by parents or persons with autism that may be useful in describing, picturing, and relating to autism. Even similar books about Asperger's syndrome will likely contain information helpful in discussing autism.

Be certain to frame any discussion about autism in the context of human differences and strengths—we are all more alike than different, and that's what makes us unique. Human beings have many gifts and talents, and some people are better at certain things than others. Be sure to highlight areas in which your child excels, balanced by gently discussing ways in which he may need to work harder because he thinks, learns, moves, or processes information differently than most people—but he is valued nonetheless. Discuss your own strengths and shortcomings (again, it may be best to do this visually in pictures, photographs, and words) and those of persons close to your child. The world needs every one of us in it in order to be whole and complete!

What is the best way to talk about autism with my child's siblings?

As a parent, all of your children potentially model a tone that *you* set. When you set a positive example, your children are poised to reflect it back, not just in how they perceive their sibling with autism, but in how they project attitudes about people with differences throughout their lives. You can include your child's siblings in a dialogue about our collective differences and similarities. You may also wish to consider the following:

- Decide if it's best to discuss autism with each of your children individually or as a family.
- Encourage your children to identify their strengths, gifts and talents, and the areas in which they have to exert more effort to

succeed or maintain.

- Talk about autism in terms of a natural experience—not something that's contagious or something that could suddenly happen to your other children.
- Pity no one, and don't make your other children believe they should feel sorry for their sibling with autism, though their future interactions may require sensitivity and compassionate accommodation.
- Don't impose unfair or unrealistic expectations on your other children by making them feel they are responsible for perpetual caretaking.
- Discuss the new ways in which the whole family will be supporting your child with autism to grow, learn, and socialize as typically as your other children.
- Think about how to include all of your children in activities designed for your child with autism—therein lie lots of playful, bonding opportunities.
- Make yourself available to answer questions now and in the future, and, if you don't have the answer, partner with your children to research it.
- Finally, be clear in setting the conditions about personal disclosure: where, when, and with whom your child's autism is or *is not* discussed.

Some family members don't believe my child's autism diagnosis. How do I handle this?

This depends on how much you value those family members, and how much time and effort you wish to expend convincing them of the truth. It may be frustrating or offensive to think someone who is not *you*, your child's parent, disbelieves his diagnosis. Depending on how discipline has been handled in families, some parents have been made to feel that their child simply requires the strict enforcement of a swat on the rear end to shape up. Remember, too, that some family members may be operating from fear of the unknown based on autism myths and stereotypes; or they may be considering how they were raised and thinking that diversity in *anyone*—let alone individuals with autism—should be kept out of sight or restricted to segregated environments.

To help you decide how to handle this situation, consider the following:

- Are these family members fearful of the stigma associated with autism?
- Do you see them often enough to make educating them otherwise a priority?
- Can they be expected to honor selective disclosure?
- Can they see beyond labels to value the beauty and wisdom your child has to offer?
- Can you react firmly yet gracefully in lieu of complaints, misinformation, and expressions of hopelessness?
- Are you willing to risk exclusion from family events if they are unwilling to yield?

Your advocacy on behalf of your child will prevail in the face of adversity, regardless of the outcome.

Since getting my child's diagnosis, and doing a lot of reading and research, I'm realizing that a lot of the information about the traits of autism is shared by my spouse. Is this possible?

This is a question that must be addressed delicately. While there is no one single-known cause for autism, among the prevailing theories is that genetics plays a part in influencing someone's predisposition to autism. You may well be seeing traits in your spouse that are similar to those in your child. You may also recognize such similarities in family lineage on both sides. Was there an uncle who wasn't very social and kept to himself, called a "hermit?" Or a cousin that would spontaneously flap his hands when he got really excited?

Your challenge is whether to share these finding with your spouse, or merely tuck them away and keep them to yourself. This is purely a personal decision based on how well you know your spouse and how well you know yourself. If you choose to reveal your suspicions, it is recommended that you do so in a private and respectful way; it would be hurtful to unexpectedly blurt out accusatory words with harmful intent in the heat of an argument (i.e., "It's your fault Bryan's autistic!"). Have you been sharing what you've been learning about autism with your spouse as you, yourself, uncover it? If so, is he receptive to it? Or do you perceive him to be resistive? Is your sense that his discomfort might stem from an unwillingness to confront the truth? On the other hand, such knowledge—if lovingly presented—may offer tremendous relief and understanding for your spouse. It is not unusual for people in their twenties, thirties, forties, and older to have high-functioning autism or Asperger's syndrome and be undiagnosed. Use what you are learning about your child and his way of being, thinking, and receiving and processing information to approach your spouse in the same manner, if you choose to.

Will my child ever need to be reevaluated in the future?

As your child is growing, learning, and developing, she may acquire new skills or may appear to slip behind other children in certain areas. If you have questions or concerns about your child's development that you think would be better resolved through a reevaluation, you can arrange for it by contacting the doctor who conducted the original evaluation or another qualified professional. (Depending on the timeframe between evaluations, your insurance may not cover a new evaluation in whole or in part.)

On occasion, because of differences in clinical perception and interpretation, a child initially diagnosed with autism may, on reevaluation, receive a new diagnosis. The new diagnosis may remain among those on the autism spectrum, or may be another commonly associated diagnosis, as previously mentioned. If your child was originally diagnosed with high-functioning autism or with PDD-NOS, a follow-up evaluation is recommended in consultation with your child's doctor. If your child appears to significantly regress, or lose previously acquired skills, such as speech or self-care abilities, a follow-up evaluation should be scheduled as soon as possible.

Chapter 3

COMMUNICATION

- If my child doesn't talk by the age most kids do, is he autistic?
- Why doesn't my child make eye contact when I talk to her?
- So, what should I do if I speak to my child and she doesn't look at me?
- What is preventing my child from talking?
- What is the most essential information that my child who doesn't talk would want me to know?
- Is there anyone who can help my child talk?
- Is there anything I should be doing to encourage my child to talk?
- Should I teach my child sign language?
- What is PECS?
- What is AAC?
- What is facilitated communication?
- Should I stick with one method of communicating with my child?
- How will I know if a communication method is working?
- Why does my child rarely talk but sings to certain songs?
- Why does my child speak, but refuses to talk to new people?
- What do I do about my child's habit of repeating things that characters in video games, commercials, and cartoons say?
- Why does my child keep asking me the same things over and over again?
- Why does my child look at me, confused, when I ask him to shake a leg and hurry up?
- How is it that my child can read and pronounce words most adults can't?
- I read that many autistic people "think in pictures." What does that mean?
- How can I best communicate with my child?
- Why does my child engage in aggressive, destructive behaviors that he knows will cause him to lose things or experiences that he likes, and that he knows are bad choices?
- How do I explain my child's eccentric behavior and tantrums to other parents in a way that shows respect to my child?
- Why did my child speak more when he was two years old than he does now at age twelve?
- What if my child never talks?

If my child doesn't talk by the age most kids do, is he autistic?

Not necessarily, no. Your child may have a speech delay without being autistic. While it's true that experiencing challenges in speaking or speaking reliably may be linked to autism, this delay alone does not make your child autistic.

Is there a family history of others who started talking later than their siblings or peers? Confer with your pediatrician before drawing any conclusions. Your child may simply need a "jump-start" in the form of occupational therapy, speech therapy, music therapy, or play activities to engage him and motivate him to begin articulating speech.

Why doesn't my child make eye contact when I talk to her?

A hallmark trait in those with autism is difficulty making or maintaining eye contact. And typically, when *anyone* doesn't look at us when we're speaking to them we automatically assume they're not listening.

But more than a few adults with autism have expressed that making eye contact is extremely challenging due to being visually distracted. In short, if your child is compelled to maintain direct eye contact, she may not be hearing a word, but if your child appears not to be listening, she is most likely absorbing nearly everything you are saying.

So, what should I do if I speak to my child and she doesn't look at me?

When the child with autism doesn't make eye contact, you may be tempted to say, "*Look at me.*" Or, you may physically take hold of your child's chin and maneuver it so that you are eye to eye. Many adults with autism have described how unpleasant and disrespectful this feels. Please discontinue the practice of grabbing hold of your child's flesh; if she, suddenly and without warning, reached out and grabbed you in precisely the same manner, you'd be tempted to quickly label it as a "behavior" and an act of physical aggression!

Making eye contact in conversation is one of our cultural mores that connotes attention and respect—but how is your child with autism supposed to know that if it hasn't been *taught?* (You'll probably need to demystify the concept of handshaking in the same way!) Explain why others expect eye contact in certain situations and discuss strategies to cope, such as looking in someone's direction as they speak, approximating eye contact by facing someone and looking at his or her earlobe or mouth, or maintaining fleeting glances interspersed with gazing away.

Once you've done that, assume that she's hearing you; but if you're still uncertain or uncomfortable you can:

- Ask her to momentarily stop what she's doing.
- Explain that you're requesting her to listen, and this is one way you can tell if she is.
- Ask clarifying questions about what you've just communicated to make certain she's got it.
- Ask her to repeat what you've just said.
- If your child doesn't talk, request that she show you in other ways that she heard and understood.
- Request that she practice giving the illusion of eye contact with you during the moment and in a natural situation.

Your child's verbal responses or physical actions will assure you that your message has been received despite a deceiving exterior.

What is preventing my child from talking?

If your child isn't talking because of a speech delay, it may be that your child's neurology simply isn't wired for speech. This is not to suggest that speech and music therapy would not prove beneficial in aiding your child to express verbal communications. But can you accept that he may *never* speak? A number of parents lament never being able to hear their child say, "I love you." However, your child is surely communicating to you in many other ways, including expressions of love.

On occasion, some individuals with autism do not begin speaking until well beyond typical developmental milestones; some who cannot speak can sing beautifully and articulately (music is lifeblood to the vast majority); still others *choose* to remain silent because they have been treated disrespectfully by those unpresuming of their intellect.

If your child does not speak, it is your job to exhaust all other alternatives to speech to find another "voice" for your child to use to express himself. It is not acceptable to believe that, because your child doesn't talk, he has nothing of value to contribute. Your child will guide you to the communication mode that works best for him after you've offered a variety of options. It is a process, and one that may require patient trial and error.

What is the most essential information that my child who doesn't talk would want me to know?

That he's smart and that he loves you.

Is there anyone who can help my child talk?

No one can promise or guarantee that they can help your child talk, but if your child is able to make the necessary neurological connections that will enable verbal speech, it will be because of your loving, patient, and consistent efforts. You may wish to consult a speech therapist or an occupational therapist. Speech therapy may aid your child in acquiring language skills or building on any verbalizations he currently makes. Occupational therapy may support your knowledge of how your child's fine-motor skills are hindering him from articulating language. Music therapy can make acquiring new language a pleasing experience through song and rhythm.

Your child will require an individualized program designed to meet his needs in order to learn verbal communication. However, a weekly or twice-weekly, one-on-one session with a specialized therapist is not enough; you will wish to partner with any therapist with whom your child interacts so as to embed elements of what they convey throughout your child's day in all that he does. In this manner, exerting his will to communicate occurs naturally within the flow of all daily routines. Narrate everything you do, see, and engage in with your child; highlight the humor and beauty in your encounters. Even if your child never communicates verbally, your lives will both be richer for the experiences you've shared.

Is there anything I should be doing to encourage my child to talk?

Two things: Identify your child's most passionate interests, and allow her the opportunity to reciprocate by teaching *you*. The chapter on valuing passions (Chapter 7) will provide you with much detail about your child's area(s) of special interest—a topic or subject of which she is absolutely enamored. Offering a new and different alternative to speech, or a new way of learning language, is a seduction of sorts; what you're offering has to be so compelling that your child will be motivated to give it a try. What better motivator than to build on something she already loves and is fascinated by?

Reciprocation should be embedded in *every* teaching and learning opportunity your child is offered. Children with developmental differences tend to be perceived as the constant recipients of all that we have to contribute in our wisdom and professional expertise—but how often are those same children permitted to give back of themselves? Rarely. Through teaching *you* how to create, operate, imitate, or play, your child will feel empowered in a way that may lead to an increased desire to communicate verbally.

Should I teach my child sign language?

The use of sign language within families can be very useful and may significantly decrease your child's (and your own) frustration level. Verbally identifying the sign paired with the sign itself can also be a technique to elicit language from your child. In addition to the essentials ("yes," "no," "drink," "eat," "toilet"), you'll want to impart signs for your child to communicate more complex wants, needs, and desires such as obtaining something or contacting someone outside of his immediate environment. You'll also want to work on conveying signs that reflect emotions so that your child can become better attuned to what he's feeling in the moment, or describe his feelings, so that his behaviors don't get misinterpreted.

Although sign language definitely has its place in the family unit and should be preserved, be cautious about limiting your child to sign language as his exclusive means of communicating because it is not universally understood. It also means that everyone with whom your child interacts *for the rest of his life* must be as fluent in sign language as he is, or you risk doing a huge disservice to him. Your child is autistic, not deaf; and even within the Deaf community there are splintered factions of individuals who use variations of standardized sign language, even "sign slang" or shorthand. To traverse his life, your child's modes of communication will require a more eclectic array of options than sign language alone.

What is PECS?

PECS is the acronym for Picture Exchange Communication System, which is based on the understanding that many people with autism are visual thinkers and learners. PECS involves creating a visual library for your child using small, manageable, and portable imagery that she may access at will in order to initiate communication. Parents, often paired with supportive professionals, have created binders, file boxes, and picture boards filled with images pertinent to the lives of their child in order to enhance communication (and prompt verbal speech), offer their child communication choices, challenge their child to discriminate between images, and promote independence in communication to the greatest extent possible. In presuming intellect, it's also best if all imagery is paired with words, or, if you know your child can read, consists of words alone. PECS can also be used to arrange visual sentences for your child to initiate or complete, such as "I want…"

PECS has been very successful for many persons with autism, but most advocate the use of real photographs or magazine clippings instead of hand-drawn or computer-generated icons, which can be confusing and subjective in their interpretation. PECS is a terrific start to fostering independence in communication but be mindful that it can be limiting; that is, it can be limited to the parameters we've set for what concepts we *think* someone desires to communicate. PECS cannot possibly capture all that someone is wondering (one young boy with autism wrote that his PECS binder "does not help me learn about life"), but it is an excellent bridge to acquiring communication skills for many.

For further information about PECS, its origins and founders, and current news, visit www.pecs.com.

What is AAC?

AAC is the acronym for Augmentative and Alternative Communication (also known as Augmentative and Assistive Communication). AAC refers to any alternative device your child may employ to supplement or augment spoken communication. This may range from the very low-tech techniques such as PECS, picture boards, picture schedules, alphabet boards, and literacy learning aids, to high-tech, sophisticated devices such as computers and computer programs with electronic storage and retrieval systems designed to suggest communication choices and activities. These could be laser pointers operated by eye gaze or muscle movements, or portable keyboards with display screens and "voice" output. (*Note:* Make certain it's programmed with a same-aged, same-sex voice, not that of an adult or, worse yet, the opposite gender.) Such available electronic devices can "speak" in response to selections entered on a keyboard or other methods controlled with motions as simple as the press of a button, a breath of air, or a furrowed brow.

AAC technology has benefited individuals with a variety of conditions that may impair the ability to produce speech, such as autism, Down syndrome, deafness, cerebral palsy, ALS or Lou Gehrig's disease, multiple sclerosis, stroke, Parkinson's, and Alzheimer's. Some parents fear that AAC will preclude or prevent their child with autism from talking by creating dependency. Please know that your child is keenly aware that everyone around him speaks, and he is striving to fit in. In other words, **AAC users who speak or have some verbal command don't abandon speech in favor of using a device!** Speech may, indeed, become increased and of greater quality, leading to improved social interactions. As is true of any technique offered as an alternative to speech, the outcome of employing an AAC device should be to enhance your child's quality of life through fostering independence in communication.

You may learn more about AAC, the wide variety of low- and high-tech devices available, and the many companies that produce AAC technology by doing an Internet search for "Augmentative and Alternative Communication."

What is facilitated communication?

Facilitated communication (FC) is a technique that builds from the premise that your child with autism is literate but unable to articulate speech in order to demonstrate his true competence. FC involves providing physical support to an individual's hand to aid him in developing confidence and motor-planning capabilities by finger-pointing to discriminate between objects, words, pictures, and icons, or to type fluently on a keyboard. When applied properly, the facilitator does not guide the person's hand, but provides *upward* resistance as the individual pushes downward to point to the object, word, picture, icon, or keyboard to complete the intended communication, before gently pulling the hand back upward prior to the next selection. It should feel something like arm-wrestling. Because the goal of FC is independence in communication free from physical support, touch at the hand should eventually be faded to the wrist, forearm, elbow, or shoulder.

The credibility of FC has been called to task in the past, and many professionals have dismissed it because there are studies that have disproven FC; they have shown it to be the result of the facilitator consciously or unconsciously moving the individual's hand to type communication that was attributed to the individual alone. Some other inconsistencies have been due to an individual's processing delay in responding to a request, or an individual singling out a background detail when a facilitator is discussing prominent items in a picture. Little known, though, are the studies that have validated FC as a viable and boundless communication alternative when used properly; and persons with autism such as Sue Rubin, Amanda Baggs, and Jamie Burke, who have progressed to independent typing, are challenging old beliefs about FC's questionability.

In the United States, the premiere resource center for FC is the Facilitated Communication Institute at New York's Syracuse University. For further information, visit http://suedweb.syr.edu/thefci.

Should I stick with one method of communicating with my child?

Do you communicate in just one way? If you think about it, you'll quickly tally up dozens of nonverbal ways in which you convey information throughout each day. When approaching how best to support the child with autism who doesn't speak, many professionals advise a "total communication" approach. This means offering your child a range of communication options simultaneously or in planned succession, and may include any or all the communication concepts reviewed thus far. These options should be integrated throughout the day, and should be used consistently by all who interact with your child. If your child cannot tell you which method is the best fit, it may make sense to provide your child with a variety of methods as opposed to limiting her to just one in the hopes that it will click for her. As your child demonstrates proficiency for one or more communication styles, those that are less used may be faded out in favor of developing and emphasizing those that appear to be most compatible for her.

How will I know if a communication method is working?

As previously suggested, your child will guide you to what makes sense for her—you'll know quickly enough what doesn't work due to the swiftness of her abandonment. You will know a communication alternative is working if your child's stress decreases and her abilities to manage and cope increase, because her communications are being heard and honored. Any communication technique that creates more work for you and your child, does not fit within the flow of your daily routines, or is not effective, reliable, and universally understandable to your child is not likely to be helpful in the long term.

How come my child rarely talks but will sing to certain songs?

The secret lies in the magic that is music! It may be that music awakens a part of the brain that induces pleasure and sheer enjoyment, triggering internal brain–body connections leading to speech otherwise dormant. Pair music with a favored activity, and you've got an unbeatable combination that may lead to enhanced articulation. Even if your child echoes lyrics or vocalizes indiscernible sounds to music, this is an important opportunity that should be seized.

You may wish to tap the expertise of a strong music therapist to learn about ways to draw out more verbalizations from your child using music. This may include the concept of "call and response," such as singing a portion of a round-robin song like "Row Your Boat" with the expectation that your child join in; or it could be a matter of gently slowing the music tempo as your child sings so as to emphasize enunciation. Remember the prior recommendation to narrate everything you do? Try this but by *singing* everything you do. You probably already know your child's favorite music or musical artists—start there, and generalize music therapy techniques throughout the day.

How come my child speaks but refuses to talk to new people?

This is likely more an issue of comfort level than it is a concern about verbal communication. If meeting someone new creates some mild anxiety for you, imagine how your child must feel. You're probably going to prompt an adverse reaction in your child if you pressure her into speaking to a stranger before she's ready—and not until she's processed everything there is to absorb about this person.

Once your child is feeling comfortable and less anxious, you should see a greater willingness to respond with verbal speech. This, in particular, may apply to meeting new therapists, educators, and clinical and medical staff of all sorts. If your child can handwrite or type, start by allowing her to reply to inquiries from strangers in this passive format.

If your child repeatedly refuses to talk with a specific person and, in addition, exhibits a strong behavioral reaction, consider the possibility that your child has experienced a traumatizing event in the presence of this individual (or someone that resembles him or her) or associates this person and his or her environment with great unpleasantness.

What do I do about my child's habit of repeating things that characters in video games, commercials, and cartoons say?

Some parents and professionals might see this as a detrimental nuisance to be extinguished. Foremost, be thankful your child with autism is saying *anything*; the child who is attempting to talk understands that the world best accommodates those who speak. Second, try re-envisioning this attribute as a strength. Many kids with speech and language delays echo or repeat what they hear on television or from people. You may even hear this referred to as *echolalia*. If your child is repeating entire lines of dialogue or phrases from movies and television, you may hear this referred to as "movie talk" or scripting (more on this in Chapter 10). Both echoing and scripting are terrific building blocks from which to cultivate functional spoken language.

A good speech therapist may be a valuable resource to you in providing strategies for making practical use of your child's repetitive speech throughout each day. You may also wish to chart the words or phrases your child is saying and create a second corresponding column in which you teach a new phrase to begin using that holds the same meaning. For example, try equating "To infinity and beyond!" with something a bit more universally understood, like "Gotta get going!" Stay-at-home parents often immediately recognize repeated words or phrases from having overheard the videos their child replays regularly; but, even in company that won't recognize these catch phrases, is there any harm in it if your child is using such language to gain confidence in breaking the ice with new people, or in identifying when a certain phrase might be appropriate to a given social situation? It may even create humor and acceptance—we *all* use certain catch phrases that share social familiarity, like "Go ahead make my day!" or "I'll be back!"

If your child repeats a word or phrase almost as a mantra (what some may call *stimming*), it may be a coping mechanism to quell anxiety or to decompress (more on this in Chapter 4).

Why does my child keep asking me the same things over and over again?

This likely has little to do with a speech concern and more to do with the idea expressed in the preceding answer: needing to quell and contain anxiety by hearing or repeating the same thing over and over. It may also be attributed to the fact that, oftentimes, children must rely on the adults in their lives for information about what's coming next, what to expect, and what is expected of them. This alone can cause tremendous issues of nervousness and anxiety.

Instead of verbally repeating your answer in reply to your child's repeated questioning (which is likely to exacerbate your patience), sit with her and write down the question *and* the answer on paper. Make the response as detailed as it needs to be in order to satisfy your child's need for information. That will aid her in feeling safe, comfortable, and in control.

Why does my child look at me, confused, when I ask him to shake a leg and hurry up?

Because in asking him to hurry up you've told him to "shake a leg," and he's interpreting what you've said *literally*. This is an example of the very literal, direct, and concrete way in which so many individuals on the autism spectrum think. They are not usually privy to the subtle nuances of social idioms that others pick up naturally, such as sarcasm, innuendo, double-entendre, slang, and irony. Instead, they often say what they mean and mean what they say—and expect you to do the same, unless you explain it otherwise. In reflecting on her need to be more conscientious in communicating with her son, one mom said, "These are things that over the years he has had to learn. Once I explain what I really mean, he then understands. When he was younger I imagine I confused him often!" In interacting with your child, be conscious of how often such figures of speech creep into your everyday conversation—you'll be surprised!

How is it that my child can read and pronounce words most adults can't?

Many adults with autism report the ability to read at an unusually early age; others say they became literate by acting like a sponge and soaking up everything around them, teaching themselves how to read when others were *unpresuming of their intellect*.

In very young children, the ability to read and pronounce complex language, such as formal or technical terms (medical terminology or the official names given to dinosaurs, for example), is called *hyperlexia*. This ability, however, doesn't mean the child understands the meaning of the word or the context in which it is most appropriately used. This can be taught, however, and the accomplishment of reading in any form is something to validate, praise, and nurture to fruition.

I read that many autistic people "think in pictures." What does that mean?

As noted previously, many—but not all—people with autism think in ways that are very visual. This often means thinking in streams of imagery such as pictures and movies, and assigning words an image from their mental "catalog" of pictures. It may sound like hard work for you because you may not be a visual thinker (you *can* do it though, with some effort, if someone directs you to "picture this" or "imagine this"), but for the person who thinks this way naturally it is an effortless and fluid process. It does, however, require that we allow the picture-thinker enough process time to match our words with their inventory of images.

How can I best communicate with my child?

Given the preceding explanation, if you wish to communicate with your child clearly and concisely in ways that will be understood and retained, ensure that you are not relying solely on verbal communication but are reinforcing your spoken words with visuals. (For the child who is more auditory than visual, you can tape record what you need to communicate so it can be replayed repeatedly at will.)

Please know that, for the picture-thinker, your spoken words evaporate and dissipate into thin air immediately after you've uttered them. (This probably accounts for the reason why a lot of children struggle in school when given exclusively verbal, didactic instruction.) Your child will be poised for failure if you give him multiple-part verbal instruction with the expectation that he reliably act on your directions—you're on step 4 or 5, and he's still on step 1 trying to match mental imagery with what you're talking about so that he can retain it. Without your cognizance of this essential principle of autism, you are wide open to misperceptions and misunderstandings about your child's abilities, and your child's self-esteem is at risk of being undermined for the self-blame he may place on himself for not being able to communicate.

Reinforcing your directions in simple, written, bulleted or numbered sequential steps will cause you to be more conscious of communicating clearly, and will aid your child in successfully interpreting your expectations of him. Unless you recognize that your child processes information best by auditory means, underscoring your communications in ways that are written, pictorial, and visual is advisable.

Why does my child engage in aggressive, destructive behaviors that he knows will cause him to lose things or experiences that he likes, and that he knows are bad choices?

Here is an instance in which to reinterpret your child's "behavior" as communication. What is transpiring for your child may be the result of several possibilities. It could be a circumstance in which your child is overwhelmed and has "maxed out" his coping skills, thus surrendering to his overloaded system. It may be that, in anticipation of participating in an activity he likes, he has caused such internal anxiousness that this "feel good" sensation escalates into out-of-control turmoil because it feels *too* good. Or it may be that he is berating himself for being imperfect by deliberating doing something to deny himself a favored activity because he is undeserving for any number of reasons that may seem overblown or illogical to you but very real to him.

The concept of being overwhelmed and "maxing out" is an issue that relates to sensory sensitivities and pacing oneself, as discussed in the next chapter. Anxiety and poor self-image may be linked to mental wellness issues that will be covered in Chapter 6. What's most important in this situation is helping your child in a loving and supportive way to identify what led to his loss of control. He may be unable to put concise language to his feelings in the moment, but this debriefing is a good preventive measure and a sound habit to nurture in preparation for future such incidents.

How do I explain my child's eccentric behavior and tantrums to other parents in a way that shows respect to my child?

First of all, your child's tantrums are *communications*, not "behaviors." Think prevention instead of intervention. If you are constantly in the position of feeling the need to explain your child's way of being to other parents, you may not be focusing enough on preventive measures that will aid your child in feeling safe and comfortable and in control in a given situation such as a crowded event with lots of distractions, noise, unfamiliar smells, and an unsettling or ambiguous agenda. Again, your child is likely not able to put language to her experience in the moment and may be unable to identify her own feelings of unease as they escalate until she's caught up in the middle of it.

Ask yourself if your child's so-called eccentric habits are really something that requires explanation. If so, you may want to revisit the previous chapter about diagnosis and the principles of disclosure.

Why did my child speak more when he was two years old than he does now at age twelve?

It may be that your child is experiencing a regression in functioning. Have you noticed his diminished ability to care for himself through bathing, dressing, toileting, and feeding? If so, consult your pediatrician with your concerns. Or perhaps his decrease in speech may have something to do with being more aware of his differences when compared to his peers now that he's twelve, more so than when he was two and largely oblivious to such social comparisons.

If you've noticed your son steadily withdrawing, not only through diminished speech but also through spending more time alone, increased irritability, trouble sleeping, eating noticeably more or less, disinterest in the things he's previously enjoyed, and having difficulty concentrating, it could indicate a depression that requires your immediate attention. He's at the age when he's especially vulnerable to such mental wellness issues (more about this in Chapter 6).

What if my child never talks?

Then this is the beauty of his natural design—he's created just as intended and you can love him for it all the more. Not talking isn't the same as not having something to say, and you and your child will be better for it if you are thorough in partnering with him to explore the myriad options and opportunities that may provide him with an alternative to verbal communication. Never disbelieve that his intelligence is not intact—you'll see it just by gazing deeply into his eyes. Never cease pursuing a way for him to express himself fully and completely as the competent, amazingly gifted human being that he is.

Chapter 4

SENSORY SENSITIVITIES

- What are sensory sensitivities?
- What are common examples of autistic sensory sensitivities?
- Is there any way I can understand how my child experiences sensory sensitivities?
- What should I do to get a handle on my child's sensory sensitivities?
- My child can talk, so why doesn't she just tell me about her sensory sensitivities?
- I can't stop going into the community just so I can accommodate my child. What should I do?
- Some suggestions for hearing sensitivities would be great; earplugs don't seem to work well for us and loud noises are excruciating for my son.
- If my child has a sensory sensitivity for sound and melts down when his brother plays the radio, why will he turn up the songs he likes full blast?
- When a child has sound sensitivities, is it better to shield her from these sounds or to teach and build tolerance?
- What is sensory processing disorder?
- What is a sensory diet?
- If I don't run a hairbrush over my child's arms every day, am I a bad parent?
- Why is it that my son hates to be touched lightly (he says it hurts), yet will ask me to lie across his chest with my full weight and seems to like this deep pressure?
- Why is handwriting so difficult for my child?
- Why does my child seem to never sit still, especially when doing school-work, but can sit still in front of the computer for hours?
- How can I persuade my child to try a variety of foods when he eats the same thing every day?
- What is *stimming*?
- Why is stimming so important to so many individuals with autism?
- A lot of therapies discourage stimming; should parents do so as well?
- How can discouraging stimming have a negative impact on my child's emotional well-being and growth?
- Is there a connection or pattern in the observation that an increase in stimming seems to precede new skills, new speech, or new behaviors?
- My other children tease or provoke the sensory sensitivities of my child with autism. How can I get them to understand?

What are sensory sensitivities?

Sensory sensitivities are the uncomfortable, painful, or upsetting sensations you receive in reaction to sensory stimuli that are beyond your tolerance threshold. These sensations relate to your five senses either singularly or in combination. For example, perhaps the scent of a certain food odor or a strong perfume makes you feel nauseated or headachy, or you may have an aversion to both the sight *and* sound of a large crowd.

Until the 1994 edition of the *Diagnostic and Statistical Manual of Health Disorders* (DSM), strong sensory reaction was included among the criteria for autism. Despite its disappearance from the DSM criteria, it is still extremely common in those with autism, and most often overlooked by parents and professionals. Because of a generalized sensitivity in many individuals with autism, their senses are impacted to a far greater degree than is the average person. Children who struggle to assimilate in this way may also have the diagnosis of sensory integration disorder.

What are common examples of autistic sensory sensitivities?

Many people with autism have reported hurtful responses to the following (not all-inclusive) list of sensory sensitivities:

- *Hearing:* Babies crying, dogs barking, cars backfiring, vacuum cleaners, school bells, fire alarms, police and ambulance sirens, certain high-pitched voices, food chewing, pencil tapping, fans and ventilation systems, music other than their own, the pronunciation of select words.
- *Vision:* Too many colors or a certain color that is painful to look at, sunlight that is too bright, harsh overhead lighting such as halogen or fluorescent lights, alternating light and shadow (especially while

driving) that creates a strobe-light effect, attempting to transition from one environment to a different environment (e.g., moving from hardwood flooring to patterned carpeting).

- *Touch:* Being touched unexpectedly or from behind, being hugged, shaking hands, bathing or having hair washed, seams on socks, clothing that is too tight, clothing that is other than soft cotton, aversion to certain textures such as something too soft or too rough to the touch, or something damp and squishy like modeling clay.

- *Smell:* Certain food odors, bathroom odors, perfumes, colognes and deodorants, pet-related smells (i.e., a fish tank), cigarette smoke, cigar and tobacco scents.

- *Taste:* Certain food textures may cause gagging or vomiting, such as hard, crunchy-textured foods like carrots and celery sticks, crunchy-style peanut butter, or rubbery, slimy-textured foods like pudding, Jell-O, tapioca, jelly, or eggs.

Is there any way I can understand how my child experiences sensory sensitivities?

Yes. Think of it in terms of a severe allergic reaction that accompanies debilitating symptoms. If the preceding list prompted you to think about some of your own sensory sensitivities, take what you know to be true of yourself and bump it up a hundred degrees in intensity and you might come close to how your child perceives the same stimuli.

To understand further, have someone lead a game of "Simon Says" with you with the expectation that you must remain mute throughout *but* participate and attend fully. The catch is, while that's occurring, someone else needs to rapidly flash the lights in the room on and off at the same time another person is drowning out your leader with static and loud music from ever-changing radio frequencies. After less than a minute, you'll feel like giving up, throwing a "tantrum," or running out of the room because of the way in which your senses are being assaulted. This is how a person with sensory sensitivities may feel. If you were a child with autism and acted out those behaviors in a classroom, you'd be called "noncompliant" or a "behavior problem."

What should I do to get a handle on my child's sensory sensitivities?

Understand that your child's insistence on predictability is, in part, a need for control when everything else around her is *out of control*. Wherever possible, try to create a home environment that is stable and routine with a family schedule that is predictable.

Next, partner with your child and others who know her best to create a sensory sensitivity inventory. Do this by devising a list. On the left side of a piece of paper, list all of the sensory sensitivities you've observed in your child. Now, down a right-hand corresponding column, record the way you've seen your child react to each sensory irritant. This will aid you in clearly defining her limits for tolerance, and will give you a clearer picture of the true issues.

Lastly, assess *yourself* and encourage those persons with whom your child has close contact during her day to do the same in order to minimize sensory concerns. Here's a list of aspects worthy of consideration:

- Perfume, cologne, and the scent of hair products may be overwhelming.
- Your breath—did you just have a cigarette or cup of coffee? Did you freshen your breath or brush your teeth after eating, especially if you had strong-smelling foods?

- The fragrance of your laundry detergent—can you use a hypoallergenic, perfume-free detergent?
- Your body temperature—are your hands ice cold or sweaty and clammy feeling?
- Long hair can be a distraction if working too closely with a child—try pulling, tying, or clipping it back off your face.
- Dangling earrings or facial jewelry can be distracting.
- Tone of voice—low, smooth, calm, and even is best.
- Clothing colors—some children may have a strong reaction to certain colors.

My child can talk, so why doesn't she just tell me about her sensory sensitivities?

Many children aren't able to pinpoint their own sensory sensitivities by identifying them as such, and may not realize the source of what's triggering them to feel anxious or even aggressive. If you can't identify what's making you feel out of sorts, it's difficult to describe what's going on in words.

If your child is one of the few who *is* able to communicate to you that the overhead lights flicker too much, or the mall is too crowded and noisy, count your blessings! You have a child who is already acutely self-aware and on her way to developing self-advocacy skills in order to get her needs met *before* she succumbs to feeling overwhelmed. Work with her to further define her sensory sensitivities in order to become increasingly knowledgeable of them.

Remember that your child is working hard at meeting expectations and holding it together as best she can to avert an outburst of any kind, but also remember that the stimuli that accost her sensory sensitivities are usually unpredictable.

I can't stop going into the community just so I can accommodate my child. What should I do?

Real life dictates that we all need to leave our homes and access our community on some occasions, if not daily. As an adult, you—more often than not—have more control over that and how it will transpire than a child does. Is your family one that is in a constant state of flux with community-based errands, chores, and activities in which your child with autism is expected to participate or tag along?

We routinely set children with autism up for failure when we are not mindful of their acute, oftentimes painful, sensory sensitivities. Your child may willingly agree to participate or accompany you in all your community-based endeavors without realizing his own personal limitations—or because he wants to please you by consenting. When numerous community activities are layered in quick succession (the mall, out to eat, grocery shopping) without consideration for your child, there is a greater likelihood that— depending on the environments—his tolerance will "max out" and he will react strongly and in ways that ultimately cause him to become undone publicly. Partner with your child to better plan, or stagger, the ways in which you access the community so that your outings are more manageable and less stressful.

Some suggestions for dealing with hearing sensitivities would be great; earplugs don't seem to work well for us and loud noises are excruciating for my son.

Earplugs might be ideal, but all too often children with autism can't tolerate accepting anything foreign into their ear canal. Besides, they don't know any other kids who wear earplugs, thus earplugs have great potential to single out and stigmatize your child as "different." However, your child *does* know lots of other kids who use light-weight headphones, like those used with an iPod, which are accepted as the norm and even cool. This may be a great coping strategy to introduce to your child—a way to filter out hurtful noises, listen to pleasing music, *and* pass for "typical" all at the same time. No one has to know that your child is using his headphones primarily to ward off distracting auditory stimuli; for all intents and purposes, he's just like any other kid grooving to his favorite music.

If my child has a sensory sensitivity for sound and melts down when his brother plays the radio, why will he turn up songs he likes full blast?

Think of it this way: was your parents' music your music? Probably not. When one of your other children is playing music they prefer, it is their music and not necessarily the music to which your child with autism chooses to listen. If you increase the volume of the nonpreferred music in direct correlation to your child's sensory sensitivities, you will understand how his brother's music is inciting agitation and distress.

The music your child turns up full blast is his music, controlled by him. However, as a parent, you have the right to dictate when, where, and how loud *all* of your children may listen to their music so as to be considerate and courteous of others—this includes your child with autism. Being autistic does not exempt you from household rules.

When a child has sound sensitivities, is it better to shield her from these sounds or to teach and build tolerance?

Part of partnering with your child may mean working together to identify specific tolerance levels on a scale of one to ten, or with images of faces experiencing sequential degrees of pain. This will reinforce the concept of identifying sensory sensitivities in a way that is direct and concrete.

Your acknowledgment of your child's sensory sensitivities—paired with your compassionate understanding that she's really trying—should promote both relief and confidence in your child. This kind of loving support may give your child the impetus and esteem she needs to try to incrementally build tolerance for certain situations and environments, or to work with you to identify some coping strategies that may provide pleasing distractions in order to lessen the intensity of the moment. More than one parent who avoided Wal-Mart discovered their child could better tolerate the environment if allowed a select amount of time in the toy department.

Applying an "all-or-nothing" approach whereby your child is expected to basically sink or swim will only result in disaster and disappointment. Collaborating with your child to slowly develop tolerance using baby steps is advised.

What is sensory processing disorder?

Sensory processing disorder is the name given to a category of sensory-based differences experienced by children with autism, as well as by those identified with learning disabilities, developmental disabilities, fragile X, ADD, ADHD, and cerebral palsy. In particular, sensory processing disorder captures subgroups specific to autism such as *sensory overresponse*, or hypersensitivity; *sensory underresponse*, or hyposensitivity; and *sensory seeking*, or craving sensory input. You may also hear these experiences referred to as *sensory integration disorder* or *sensory integration dysfunction*—the inability to assimilate or integrate input through the senses in order to organize, interpret, and respond to it in ways that are considered typical.

Children who are challenged with these types of sensory-related issues may be unable to maintain alertness, cannot contain themselves if distressed, and have difficulty with eating, sleeping, and toileting. This, in turn, impacts their ability to concentrate, participate, and learn in school, home, and community. It could manifest itself in a child's distrust of various environments, inability to stay in control, being hyperprotective of themselves, and projecting what may be labeled as overexaggerated reactions to the physical world. It is unknown if all individuals with acute sensory sensitivities, such as those associated with autism, would qualify as experiencing sensory processing disorder, but a respectful speculation would be to approach your child's sensory sensitivities in ways akin to how sensory processing disorder is supported (read on).

What is a sensory diet?

A sensory diet pertains to the proper degree, kind, and frequency of sensory experiences provided to your child to attain and maintain a level of optimal functioning. Professionals who specialize in a variety of therapies may be able to deliver a proper "sensory diet" to your child via various types of activities to aid in de-escalating or de-sensitizing your child's sensory sensitivities; or such professionals may have access to (often costly) equipment or accoutrements specially designed to integrate or enhance a pleasing sensory experience.

If you choose to solicit the aid of professionals to support your understanding of developing a sensory diet for your child, it is important to understand that the concepts *they* impart to your child should be fun and enjoyable (not enforced), and easily replicated by you *throughout* your child's typical day. It is not likely to be beneficial to your child if his therapist is the only person interacting with him in this way, and if your child is using only the therapist's specialized equipment once or twice a week.

A sensory diet should include *natural* opportunities to employ some version of therapy recommendations during play or task activities using everyday items, or toys with which your child already plays. This should also include embedding reciprocal opportunities while working on the sensory diet, like encouraging your child to take turns with his brothers and sisters to use differently textured craft materials for a family art project. Other natural examples may include following a real or imaginary recipe using differently textured ingredients; folding warm, fuzzy towels right from the dryer; applying deep pressure to body parts using sofa cushions or pillows (instead of a therapy ball); and any number of water-play games.

If I don't run a hairbrush over my child's arms every day, am I a bad parent?

Attempting to de-sensitize children by "brushing" the bristles of a hairbrush over the surface of their skin is a popular sensory integration therapy technique. But in light of the preceding information, does it meet the criteria of a natural opportunity? Not if you have to consciously schedule it or feel guilty if you don't get to it. Ask yourself, too, how many children do you know whose parents plan a time to run a hairbrush over their skin? The same or similar sensation might be embedded into your child's typical routines during the times he's dressing in the morning or taking a warm bath at night. Refusing to participate in *any* professional recommendation that does not feel right for you and your child doesn't make you a bad parent, just an intuitive one with your child's best interests at heart.

Why is it that my son hates to be touched lightly (he says it hurts), yet will ask me to lie across his chest with my full weight and seems to like this deep pressure?

Your son may be an individual who has a hyposensitive sensory system. In other words, light touch or the sensation of certain fabrics (think cashmere) will create an extreme and unpleasant reaction, but deep pressure helps him to feel reconnected to his body and limbs. Does he generally seem unaware of certain stimuli, passive or apathetic, lacking in physical agility, and require extra stimulation to pay attention? If so, you may also notice him not only wanting you to lie on him, but there may be times when he'll burrow under sofa cushions and mattresses, or self-swaddle in sleeping bags, comforters, and blankets, or even throw rugs over himself in order to achieve the same comforting sensory input.

Part of teaching self-advocacy is educating him about his own needs, and supporting him to get his needs met as independently as possible. Will he wear clothes in layers during the day, such as an undershirt, regular shirt, and sweater, and then come home and decompress in his own way? Sometimes parents and professionals give children with autism weighted vests to wear, but this can look stigmatizing if the vests don't blend well, and such vests shouldn't be worn constantly. One young boy with autism who lived in a rural setting had an older brother who regularly wore a hunting vest weighted with related gear; the boy took to wearing a similar hunting vest and blended with his peers seamlessly.

There are times when we all feel better wrapped up in a comforter or getting a prolonged bear hug from someone who cares for us— remember, we are all more alike than different.

Why is handwriting so difficult for my child?

Lots of people on the autism spectrum have difficulty handwriting in ways that are clear and legible (but then, so do many doctors). This is known as *dysgraphia*. It is the inability to produce discernible handwriting, and may include elements of dyslexia due to numbers and characters being reversed, out of sequence, or written upside down. In the child with autism, it may be attributed to challenges making adequate brain–body connections in general (especially as it pertains to fine-motor skills such as handwriting or properly grasping silverware), or it could result from language-processing difficulties such as not enough processing time, thinking too far ahead, or not being able to keep up with verbal instruction.

One strategy that may be helpful is to have your child practice handwriting in a stress-free, pressure-free environment, and suggest she write about a topic of great interest to her. This way, you'll be able to note the greater care she is (or still isn't) able to invest in her handwriting, and get a sense for the kind of processing time she requires to produce quality handwriting. Other strategies may include using different kinds of ruled paper, allowing additional time for tests, and removing expectations that work is graded "for neatness."

Fortunately, beyond school years, no one nowadays is required to handwrite much of anything! Everyone types at a keyboard, and the child who struggles with dysgraphia may compensate brilliantly on the computer. If your child types well, but doesn't have good handwriting, advocate that such an adaptation be made in school. One mom worked with her son's educators to find compromise, and said: "We have finally been given the accommodation to allow him to type most of his schoolwork. He is ten and can now type faster than me."

Why does my child seem to never sit still, especially when doing schoolwork, but can sit still in front of the computer for hours?

Have you taken careful note of *what* she's doing in front of the computer for hours? It's likely something very pleasing, if not something directly related to her most passionate of interests. Or is she socializing by emailing or instant messaging friends?

There may be other reasons why your child has attention issues in school but can focus on the computer at home. Foremost, when considering sensory sensitivities, there are likely far fewer distractions or hurtful stimuli in the home environment than during the school day. Looking forward to a time to "decompress" while immersed in using the computer may be your child's way of coping.

If she struggles to focus while doing schoolwork or homework, it may be because she doesn't understand what's expected, it hasn't been clearly explained, or it doesn't challenge her intellect and she's bored by it. If your child's intellect is not presumed in school, she may be given schoolwork that is below her peers' grade level; or, she may just associate schoolwork with an unpleasant learning environment. You'll read more about creating incentives to "demystify" hard-to-understand schoolwork concepts in Chapter 7, Valuing Passions.

How can I persuade my child to try a variety of foods when he eats the same thing everyday?

Eating only a very limited diet is a common experience among children (and even adults) with autism; many have a very sensitive palate and can only tolerate certain taste sensations and textures. Many adults with autism who were forced to eat foods before they were ready now complain of experiencing unpleasant food issues or eating disorders; on the flip side, parents complain that their child with autism practically lives on chicken nuggets and French fries, for example, and nothing else!

This is an area where you may wish to be mindful of choosing your battles, especially if your child is not losing weight and if he'll take a daily multivitamin in some form. This doesn't mean you shouldn't continue offering all the good foods you want your child to try—just maybe not a full serving on the same plate and definitely *not* touching the other foods. You'll also wish to examine your own eating habits—do you practice what you preach, or have you set an unfavorable example? You can't eat what's not there (i.e., what you don't buy), and your child's food preferences are acquired tastes from the choices you've provided.

One savvy professional has a smell it–lick it–taste it policy of intervention. That is, she will make it clear that a child does not have to eat an undesired food, but will recommend it be introduced incrementally. If the scent is acceptable, then the child is encouraged to lick it; if it passes muster after that, the child is encouraged to try a small mouthful (don't many typical adults do the same thing when offered certain hors d'oeuvres?). You may also find that the child will autism will venture out, on his own, and try a new food taste when he's ready; be prepared to be taken completely by surprise when it happens—it'll likely be by sampling a portion of what's already on your plate!

What is *stimming*?

Stimming, or *self-stimulatory behavior,* is the oftentimes constant, repetitive actions or activities in which someone with autism may engage. To list just a few, these actions or activities may include:

- twirling a piece of string or rope;
- flicking a light switch on and off;
- spinning an object such as a coin, wheel on a toy, or plastic lid;
- flickering one's fingers;
- hand flapping;
- verbally repeating a word, phrase, or vocalization;
- physically rocking or twirling;
- opening and closing a door; and
- turning a faucet on and off.

Just as there's an "inside" culture among persons with autism who affectionately call one another *auties* or *Aspies,* it is also considered acceptable for that culture to refer to the above activities as *stims,* *stimmies,* or *stimming.* However, anyone outside of that culture is encouraged to adopt a new, more respectful language by describing these activities as *self-soothing* or *self-regulating* actions or activities—not behaviors.

Why is stimming important to so many individuals with autism?

Self-soothing or self-regulating actions or activities are not mindless, purposeless behaviors. In fact, they have a very real purpose as individual coping mechanisms and survival tactics. As such, self-soothing and self-regulating actions and activities are a strength, employed most often by individuals who are feeling overwhelmed in response to their environment and are trying to maintain control. Solace is found in the safety of the *sameness* of the repetition of the action, which is controlled by the individual. Bear in mind that, for those with autism, there is safety in sameness and a comfort in that which is familiar. You may receive similar solace by repeatedly rubbing your hands, shaking your leg, twirling a piece of hair, or toying with a piece of jewelry.

A lot of therapies discourage stimming; should parents do so as well?

You may notice that your child's need to engage in self-soothing or self-regulating actions and activities increases in intensity when he's feeling *a lot* of something—a lot happy and excited, or a lot anxious and upset. Again, this is your child's way of coping and trying to maintain control. You may wish to partner with your child to augment or gradually attempt to supplant these activities, but your child may always have the need to engage in the thing that helps him to feel safe, comfortable, and in control.

Options to consider include empowering your child to identify and communicate his environmental triggers and irritants so that adaptations and accommodations may be made; or offering your child a "secret weapon" in the form of a small, personal object that relates to someone or something very important that your child can keep tucked away in his pocket and take comfort in knowing it is there when times get stressful. (This is similar to your wearing a cross or wedding band, or keeping photos of your children and family in your purse or on your desk.)

How can discouraging stimming have a negative impact on my child's emotional well-being and growth?

If you choose to view your child's self-soothing or self-regulating actions and activities as autistic stereotypes, as detrimental or stigmatizing, and you pursue the course of extinguishing them behaviorally, you may well succeed—but it is nearly guaranteed that something else will immediately surface to replace it, and that might be a "something else" you hadn't bargained on—such as a self-injurious action or activity, like head banging or hitting one's face.

It's important to realize that, as an adult, you may find yourself in virtually any environment that causes you distress and discomfort, but you have the option of communicating an excuse to exit the unsettling environment, even if only temporarily, by simply stating "Please excuse me" and getting up to leave. Unless you teach your child with autism this concept, she will not realize that she has the same option available to her as well; she will feel compelled to remain in the environment no matter how overwhelming it's become. Eventually, she will exhaust her coping strategies and melt down. We are then poised to lay blame by labeling what just transpired as behavioral, disruptive, noncompliant, or even physically aggressive.

Lots of children with autism are amazingly gifted in having discovered the self-soothing option themselves—they're the kids who are constantly asking to go to the bathroom during the day; it's not because they need to go to the bathroom, it's because they need a *break* in order to pace themselves (more on this in the school success chapter, Chapter 11). Instead of extinguishing "stimming," look at what's fair and seek a resolution that's a compromise.

Is there a connection or pattern in the observation that an increase in stimming seems to precede new skills, new speech, or new behaviors?

An increase in self-soothing or self-regulating actions and activities is definitely occurring in reaction to *something*. It may be that your child is responding to internal changes that are occurring that he can sense but over which he hasn't much control. This may be an exciting and scary experience, and might be reflected in his outwardly processing what is transpiring internally by intensifying his need to feel safe and comfortable and in control.

If you are seeing positive changes take place after such activities— for example, your child acquires new verbal language—just continue to monitor behavior and attitudes. If you are seeing a deterioration of skills in terms of behavior that seems to be communicating distress or a loss of control, you may be advised to consult with a neurologist—the increase in your child's need to engage in self-soothing or self-regulating actions and activities could be precursors to the onset of seizure activity, which would certainly create a sense of losing control in your child.

My other children tease or provoke the sensory sensitivities of my child with autism. How can I get them to understand?

Kids are kids, and some teasing among siblings is natural and to be expected—in addition to taking it, does your child with autism dish it out by pushing her siblings' buttons too? It's up to you to decide as a parent how much or how little you're willing to tolerate, and what constitutes good-natured ribbing that quickly blows over versus deliberate and methodical attempts to cause someone to become undone.

If you are leaning toward the latter, trust your intuition and have a sit-down powwow with your child's siblings about her sensory sensitivities. Discuss how to better relate to this degree of sensitivity by recalling past events that were unpleasant for your other children, such as intolerance for a fireworks display or the inability to eat a certain kind of food because of its temperature, taste, or scent.

You may also wish to try the "Simon Says" activity previously mentioned as another way to convey the extremes to which your child with autism experiences her world. Instead of "Simon Says," pick up one of your children's arithmetic books and quickly dictate math problems amidst flickering lights and a blaring radio. If all else fails, this little exercise should awaken her siblings to a renewed understanding—and perhaps appreciation—of the challenges she faces everyday.

Chapter 5 PHYSICAL WELL-BEING

- Why does my child bang his head against the wall and floor?
- Why does my child try to eat lint and other small inedible objects off the floor?
- What is proprioception and what does it mean for my child?
- How can physical therapy or occupational therapy help?
- What about an exercise routine for my child?
- I've heard that martial arts are good for kids with autism. Why is that?
- Why is my child fascinated by water?
- Why does my child love to play with water in the sink, but screams and resists taking a bath?
- I've heard that people with autism don't feel pain, at least not the way other people do. Is this true?
- How can I tell if my child who doesn't talk experiences pain?
- My child talks, so why isn't she telling me when something hurts?
- My child *hates* going to the doctor—could this also be why he's not reporting pain?
- How do I make trips to the dentist more bearable?
- Why does my child cry and carry on over a paper cut, but only just now told me it's been burning when she urinates for the past three days?
- How can I get my child to brush his teeth (it's always a struggle)?
- Are kids with autism prone to certain kinds of physical pain?
- What is the gluten-free and casein-free diet?
- Could my child have allergies in addition to her autism?
- Nutrition is such a huge concern when a child refuses most foods—how can I be sure my child is getting what he needs?
- My child overeats—is there anything I could or should do about it?
- I notice that my child's behavior seems to spike after eating certain foods—why is that?
- My child will urinate appropriately, but how can I get him to move his bowels in the toilet?
- How do I communicate toileting concepts to my child?
- I caught my eleven-year-old-son pulling on his penis—what should I do about this?
- How do I help my daughter with autism understand menstruation?

Why does my child bang his head against the wall and floor?

Your child with autism may be banging his head for several reasons. Foremost, however, may be his inability to communicate his own physical pain and discomfort. Do not waste any time in finding out if there's a health-related condition that has gone undetected, undiagnosed, and untreated. Head banging in children with autism has almost become acceptable as symptomatic of autism; discern it as a communication, not a "behavior" without any purpose. Oftentimes, children who do not speak or do not speak reliably are unable to put language to or otherwise communicate when something is wrong. Might it be that your child is trying to alleviate a headache or migraine, sinus pressure, an ear infection, or a dental impaction?

Your child may also be responding to hurtful sensory sensitivities. When are the times he is most likely to engage in this activity? Is it possible that he is reacting to emotional upset? Have people been unpresuming of his intellect by talking about him in front of him, or have very delicate subjects been openly discussed in his presence because it was believed it didn't matter if he overheard or not? Finally, might it be that he is hyposensitive and, by head banging, he is seeking extreme sensory input? These are all areas to be considered simultaneously, but not before exhausting the possibility that severe undiagnosed pain may be at the root of your child's communication.

Why does my child try to eat lint and other small inedible objects off the floor?

Your child is likely very detail oriented, and could probably spot a tiny piece of lint on the floor from across the room. This is may be helpful in aiding you to keep things tidy, but oftentimes it doesn't stop at merely spotting the piece of lint; unless you catch your child in the act, it usually ends up in his mouth. You will hear this kind of activity referred to as *pica behavior* or just *pica*. Obviously you don't wish for your child to put small objects he finds on the floor in his mouth for reasons of safety (a sharp or pointy object could cut him or become a choking hazard) and hygiene (you don't know what it is or where it's been).

Assess the times when your child is most likely to engage in this activity—does it seem random, or does it occur in conjunction with a situation that has caused a strong emotion? Might it be that manipulating a small object in his mouth is a self-soothing or self-regulating action and activity for your child? If so, you'll need to reassess the environments in which he's most likely to engage in this activity. Or might it be that he is seeking sensory input on his palate and between his teeth in the way that some people grind their teeth?

Try a written narrative, similar to those found at the back of this book, to explain why putting items found on the floor into your mouth is undesirable, and be clear to communicate your parental expectations that it discontinue while offering a list of alternatives. In compromise, be certain that you intervene and catch your child in the act next time; thank your child for handing over the item (before it gets to his mouth), and redirect him to something acceptable he *can* put in his mouth, such as a piece of fruit, sugarless candy, or sugarless gum. Chewing gum tends to provide the right kind of sensory feedback some kids crave. (You will know they're done if they start to toy with it and no longer wish to chew on it.)

What's proprioception and what does it mean for my child?

Proprioception is the name given to the experience common to many people with autism who feel disconnected from their limbs, or are unsure of their physical relationship within the space they occupy. Their arms, legs, fingers, and toes may feel foreign to them, or they may seem overly cautious and tenuous when walking. It may be part and parcel of the neurological blips, misfires, and disconnects in those with autism whose bodies are not properly receiving the signals the brain is sending.

To understand, try an exercise you may remember from childhood: hold both arms outstretched in front of you, and cross your hands over your wrists so that you can interlocked your fingers palm to palm. Once your fingers are interlocked, bend your arms back and inward so that your interlocked hands come up through the space that had been between your outstretched arms. Now, one at a time, try moving each of your interlocked fingers—or, better yet, have someone else indicate which finger you may move. This hit-or-miss type of "crossed wire" sensation will enable you to better understand your child's daily struggles with her own neurology.

How can physical therapy or occupational therapy help?

A physical therapist (PT) or occupational therapist (OT) may offer your child activities to facilitate a "rewiring" process in order for your child to make better sense of her body. A PT will focus on gross-motor skills such as walking, running, bending, stretching, and tumbling using the limbs; an OT's expertise is in developing the fine-motor skills required for someone to dress oneself (buttons and zippers, tie or Velcro shoes), bite and chew properly, and adeptly manipulate objects in one's fingers such as silverware, scissors, writing implements, or a computer keyboard. One or both types of therapy in combination may gain your child a better awareness of his limbs and his relationship to his surroundings.

A good therapist will work with you to determine what recommendations are easily replicated by you and your family within the context of your typical daily routines and using everyday items found in your home. Therapy activities should be interpreted by your child as play and fun, not singled out as specialized work that distinguishes him from other children. Any therapy recommendations that can be applied to play activities that include all children, regardless of ability or disability, will work best.

What about an exercise routine for my child?

We are hearing so much about childhood obesity these days, coupled with news about children's poor eating habits and lack of exercise. If your child with autism is not as graceful or as physically agile as she would wish to be, it is likely that she is sedentary as well. Your child may have already been humiliated or singled out, described as awkward and clumsy by those less sensitive. Some children with autism have an aversion to typical sports activities because they do not comprehend the concept of competition, winning and losing, and the pressure to achieve within very limited time frames.

When considering an exercise program for your child, partner with her to focus on recreational activities that are self-contained and noncompetitive. Self-contained means that the activity can occur in isolation or in the same space as other people. Noncompetitive means there is no winner or loser, and no race-to-the-finish expectation that one excel or score points. Always act on the advice of your child's pediatrician, with whom you should consult; and start low and go slow by looking at attainable, pleasurable, low-impact activities set to your child's favorite music.

Examples of self-contained, noncompetitive recreational opportunities that may provide your child with health benefits might include:

- walking,
- bike riding,
- horseback riding,

- weight training,
- jumping rope,
- dancing/aerobics,
- shooting hoops, and
- playing hopscotch.

Partners in any of these and other activities can include you and your spouse, siblings, extended family, classmates, or neighborhood children.

I've heard that martial arts are good for kids with autism. Why is that?

Martial arts, karate, judo, tai chi, tai bo, and yoga may offer your child with autism a training program that best suits her way of being and thinking: very visual, lots of repetition, sequential and incremental learning, levels of achievement designated by color (in martial arts)—all in a manner that is self-contained and noncompetitive.

Martial arts also dictates slow, deliberate, and methodical aware-ness of one's limbs as they relate to space and to one another whether in motion or holding a position; this may definitely promote a heightened brain–body awareness for your child. In addi-tion, there is no rush, and participants may progress at their own pace and comfort level. Through martial arts of one form or another, many children with autism have experienced optimized health benefits while concurrently expanding their social and personal successes.

Why is my child fascinated by water?

Being in or near water is extremely important to the vast majority of people on the autism spectrum, for reasons unknown. It may be that the endless variations of fluidity are a welcome downtime diversion for some; for others who love to swim, the buoyancy and overall pressure of water may provide much-needed sensory input, and the solitary aspects of being alone in water or underwater may be greatly pleasing.

You may notice that your child loves to play in the bathtub or take long, soothing showers. If you encourage this interest, you may find that your child takes to swimming like a fish. Large pools may be too overwhelming, however, and indoor, enclosed pools can become crowded and echoing. As was recommended with defining your child's exercise program, start low and go slow. Do not force your child into the water before he's ready. (You're sure to forever traumatize him if you pick him up and throw him in the way some of us were taught to swim.) Health experts consider swimming, exercising in water, and moving with and against its natural resistance among the very best of exercise modalities for overall physical fitness and wellness benefits.

Why does my child love to play with water in the sink, but screams and resists taking a bath?

Your child may have already discovered a fascination with water and the infinite ways in which it can be manipulated. However, if your child does not behave similarly when taking a bath, there are several possibilities to consider. It would seem as though any child who reacts this way may have had a severely unpleasant or traumatizing experience in water or with bathing. Questions to ask include the following:

- Was he not given enough time to transition into the water?
- Was the water temperature too extreme for his sensory sensitivities?
- Was he ever bathed too impatiently?
- Is he fearful of the sound of running water?
- Is he afraid of being sucked down the drain?
- Does he perceive the bathtub as an overwhelmingly huge space to occupy?

- Does he complain that hair washing is painful due to a sensitive scalp?

In reviewing these areas of concern, you'll want to partner with your child to discuss strategies and compromise, such as finding ways that he can use to assume greater control over the whole bathing experience (turning on/off the water faucet, setting the temperature, bathing himself as much as possible); making bath time pleasurable with scented water, bubbles, water toys, and washable bath crayons; or maybe looking at bathing in a smaller, more enclosed container. Once you sift through these aspects of bathing, you will soon recognize that it's not the water that is the issue, it's one or more elements of the bathing routine.

I've heard that people with autism don't feel pain, at least not the way other people do. Is this true?

This is one of those myths that's been generalized to include *all* persons with autism when, it fact, it may hold only partial application for some. You may notice that your child does not react in ways you'd expect in response to what should be a physically painful experience. This may be disconcerting, especially if your child doesn't have a reliable way to communicate in general, let alone communicate pain and discomfort. If your child has a *flat affect*, meaning her face may reflect little to no emotion, ascertaining her pain may be even more difficult.

If you perceive your child not to be responding to pain or to have a very high tolerance for pain (little to no reaction to banging his head, arms, or legs into something, for example), it may be related to improper sensory processing. Your child may be failing to assimilate internal "signals" his brain is sending his body in order to register pain. Sensory sensitivity, physical and occupational therapy, and exercise opportunities, in consultation with your child's pediatrician, may enable your child to effect the necessary brain–body connections required to detect physical pain.

How can I tell if my child who doesn't talk experiences pain?

You will need to be very attentive and vigilant by paying careful attention to your child's overall mood and demeanor—pain affects behavior! If your child cannot tell you she's in pain, and is not outwardly indicating pain in any way, it's got to come out somehow. Think about the last time you were in significant pain and discomfort from a migraine, menstrual cramping, esophageal reflux, ulcer, or a sprained limb. Now think about how moody and irritable you felt, quick to lash out at others, hypersensitive to noise or light, wanting only to lay in bed with the covers pulled up over your head.

Now magnify *your* behavior in accordance with your child's autism and you'll know to watch for unexplained or unexpected spikes in your child's behavior, changes in her appetite or sleep, or that she's more deliberate or careful dressing and undressing. You'll also need to be vigilant in surveying your child for marks, bruises, rashes, or reddened areas on your child's body. If your child can communicate "yes" or "no" in some fashion, you'll have to play twenty questions by asking "Does it hurt here … or here?"

If there have been times in your child's history when you know she's been in pain because of how she's reacted, create a pain inventory in the same way that you'd create the sensory sensitivity inventory discussed in Chapter 4 (the two will be closely intertwined). Be certain to document the ways in which your child has historically reacted to pain, or the ways in which you finally uncovered the source of her pain; such information will be of invaluable future use.

My child talks, so why isn't she telling me when something hurts?

You may find it totally disconcerting that your child is walking around in pain without saying a word—wouldn't common sense dictate otherwise? Yes, but only if you've been *taught* such social norms. One mom described her child's inability to report pain as "He accepts it as reality, and doesn't see it as something that can be changed."

There may be a number of reasons why your speaking child is not reporting pain:

- Unless it has been taught, he may not realize that there is a social and parental expectation that when you are in pain, you tell someone.
- Your child may not understand that treatment is an option, and is available in order to gain relief from what ails him.
- Your child may not realize that what he's experiencing is different than what anyone else is feeling, and so accepts it as "normal," like the boy with autism who had only just been diagnosed with mild asthma. His first words after treatment were "Mom, I didn't know it wasn't supposed to hurt when you breathe."
- Your child may be aware that something's not quite right, but is embarrassed, scared, or ashamed to confess that there's anything wrong because of a perfectionism mind-set.

In addition to partnering with your child to create a pain inventory, you'll also want to reinforce the urgent importance of properly reporting pain. You may do this visually by effecting a series of calm to grimacing faces indicating pain intensity, or develop a numerical scale by which your child can communicate degrees of pain in comparison from highest to lowest tolerance. Professionals and educators in your child's life can help you to brainstorm and implement any pain-identification system you devise.

My child *hates* going to the doctor—could this also be why he's not reporting pain?

Yes, your child may be concealing his pain out of a fear of doctors. You may have the good fortune of collaborating with some terrific doctors who understand how to be sensitive and patient in treating your child, but you may also encounter some who are not personable, and may come across as intolerant or even rough.

Your child may not only associate an unpleasant personality with your doctor, but this may also be compounded by a strange environment with unusual smells, unfamiliar faces, and uncomfortable lighting. Couple this with being examined, poked, and prodded, then magnify it through your child's autistic lens, and you may better appreciate his desire to intentionally withhold information about pain and discomfort in order to avoid such an ordeal. Read on to the next question for further insight.

How do I make trips to the dentist more bearable?

We *all* know that trips to the dentist can create lots of anxiety, nervousness, and apprehension, especially for children. If a real estate agent's mantra is "Location, location, location," yours will soon be "Prevention, prevention, prevention." Preparing to see the dentist, or any physician who has the potential to restrict your child's ability to move, absolve personal control, and inflict pain, will require lots of careful planning in advance of the appointment so that you do not surrender to the parental pitfalls of coaxing, cajoling, or threatening your child into cooperating. You'll only make an unpleasant situation worse, and your picture-thinking child with autism will likely be traumatized by instantly conjuring vivid imagery at the mere mention of the word *dentist*. In extreme circumstances, some individuals require sedation in order to receive a dental exam; you'll wish to avoid setting this precedent if possible. Here's some helpful advice that may prove useful:

- If at all possible, plan to meet the dentist and hygienist in advance of the appointment day to greet them and tour the office.
- Inform your child, using photos and other images, of exactly what to expect during the appointment.
- If your child talks, allow her to discuss her fears and concerns; if she doesn't speak, provide gentle assurances that you'll not leave her side during the procedure.
- Plan on scheduling a preferred activity immediately following the appointment and honor those plans no matter how things go during the procedure.
- Hold your child's hand, or offer her a stress ball to squeeze.
- Be certain she and the dentist understand how she'll indicate if she needs a break.
- Allow your child to listen to favorite music on headphones (which helps drown out the penetrating sound of the drill) or watch a DVD on a portable player during the exam.
- Practice taking deep breaths together to remain as calm as possible.
- Offer to gently stroke or massage your child during the procedure.

If your dentist has had experience in treating children who are very sensitive, he or she (or the hygienist) may have additional suggestions to recommend to you and your child to greatly lessen stress and make the appointment more bearable.

Why does my child cry and carry on over a paper cut, but only just now told me it's been burning when she urinates for the past three days?

Nerve endings are most sensitive in our extremities, like fingers—ever double over in excruciating pain from having stubbed your toe? Not only that, a cut is a very visual injury no matter how minor; it's an unpredictable affront to the skin's landscape that your child may find painful, distressing, and annoying enough to very nearly obsess over. A cut also comes with blood, which is exceptionally visual and, depending on your child's mental associations with blood, could cause her to manifest an extreme visceral or seemingly overexaggerated reaction. A urinary tract infection is internal—therefore, invisible—and the pain is only as temporary as the duration of time it takes to urinate, so your child may have forgotten about the momentary burning. It also may not create anywhere near the kind of reaction as a small cut for some of the reasons shared here and in the previous discussion about why pain goes unreported.

How can I get my child to brush his teeth (it's always a struggle)?

First, as a parent, you have the right to set the rules about your expectation that teeth will be brushed. Second, in what ways can you afford your child with autism as much control as possible during this process? And third, how can you make it as pleasant and pleasing as possible?

To address the first point, you'll want to—literally—spell it out by visually explaining the hows and whys of teeth brushing and the potential consequences of poor oral hygiene (not as a threat but as a reality). You'll also want to visually convey a sequence of steps for the beginning, middle, and end of the tooth-brushing process. Build tooth brushing into your family's schedule following or preceding specific activities in order to make it a predictable, known quantity.

In allowing your child some measure of control, can he select his own toothbrush and toothpaste flavor (yours may be too strong-smelling and tasting)? If he tends to gag on the toothpaste, can you apply less than you'd use? If he gags on the toothbrush, can you use one with a compact head? You may grant your child further control by recommending he count a certain number of strokes, top and bottom.

Lastly, to make it as pleasing as possible, try "sandwiching" tooth brushing between two preferred activities. Allow your child to listen to his favorite music during tooth brushing, or let him have some extra time to play in the water following the process. If your child has a doll or action figure, let him brush his toy's teeth (or yours!) too. Also try letting him brush his teeth in his bedroom, and consider an electric toothbrush with an on–off switch, a water-pic–type device, or a fingertip baby-style toothpaste applicator to start.

Are kids with autism prone to certain kinds of physical pain?

Children with autism often have very delicate digestive systems, and tend to be prone to pain and discomfort associated with gastrointestinal complications. This may manifest in severe gas and cramping, bloating, constipation, impaction, and diarrhea. The gas part may be misinterpreted as "behavioral" in nature, as may the act of rectal digging to relieve bowel impaction.

Set aside your initial interpretation of inappropriate or embarrassing "behavior" related to your child's bodily functions and rethink what's occurring in terms of the symptoms your child is trying to independently alleviate—think of it as a form of communication. For example, one young man regularly came to school, climbed up on his desktop, clutched his stomach, and screamed. His actions were treated as "behavioral noncompliance" when in fact he was experiencing a lower gastrointestinal tract bacterium that was inciting what must have been breathtaking pain. Once the problem was identified as medical in nature and he received antibiotic treatment, the "behavior" ceased. When in doubt, err on the side of caution and rule out pain as the source of your child's communications of all digestive-related concerns.

What is the gluten- and casein-free diet?

The gluten- and casein-free diet pertains to the inability experienced by some individuals on the autism spectrum to properly digest wheat and dairy-based food products. Gluten is found in most oat products in addition to those containing wheat, rye, and barley (which include all cereals, crackers, and cookies). Casein is inherent to milk, butter, yogurt, cottage cheese, cream cheese, and other cheese products.

You may have heard of "leaky gut" syndrome as related to autism. This is the process by which the proteins from these foods do not break down in the digestive system, and leak through the stomach lining into the bloodstream, eventually affecting the opiate receptors in the brain. If your child craves—thrives upon—these food items exclusively, it may be due to an addictive sensation he receives following their consumption.

The gluten- and casein-free diet operates from the premise that not only is it an important health benefit to eliminate these foods, but symptoms of autism are claimed by some to actually improve with regards to attention span, sociability, and concentration. Because gluten and casein are found in such a pervasive and diverse range of food products, many families find it extremely difficult to incorporate such a restrictive diet into their lives for the suggested three-month minimum, if not indefinitely.

To learn more about the gluten- and casein-free diet, and available wheat and dairy substitutes, start by checking out the following Internet resources in addition to a wide variety of related cookbooks: www.glutensolutions.com, www.glutenfree.com, www.gfcfdiet.com, and www.glutenfreemall.com.

Could my child have allergies in addition to her autism?

While it is estimated that three million Americans suffer from wheat allergies, and nine hundred thousand have an intolerance for gluten, it is unknown how many children with autism are affected. Remember that your child's entire being is inherently gentle. This means your child may be susceptible to other types of food allergies as well as to a broad range of additional allergens. These may include:

- smoke,
- dust,
- mold,
- mildew,
- fungus,
- air pollution,
- animal dander (cats, dogs, birds, rodents),
- fibers found in carpets,
- clothing fabrics,
- aerosol sprays, and
- plant pollen.

One child with autism was so sensitive to certain clothing fibers that he would get a severe red rash in reaction to anything other than cotton against his skin; another child had a strong aversion to her teacher and eventually someone realized the teacher's clothes always had cat hair on them! In knowing that pain affects behavior, please be very vigilant in identifying and seeking treatment of allergy symptoms in your child, such as ear infections and blockages; red, runny, itchy eyes and nose; dark circles under the eyes; swollen glands; and a sore or scratchy throat.

Nutrition is such a huge concern when a child refuses most foods—how can I be sure my child is getting what he needs?

As previously touched on in Chapter 4, many children with autism have an extremely sensitive and tactile-defensive palate that causes them anxiety over eating foods other than those with which they are comfortable taste- and texture-wise.

If your reservations persist, begin by seeking the advice of your child's pediatrician and ask for a referral to a local dietician or nutritionist. Most hospitals and medical centers have such a professional on staff, and there may be great benefit to locating someone who has had experience in strategizing and encouraging reluctant children to eat new foods.

A dietician or nutritionist should also work with you to review your child's diet and offer you suggestions for substituting, eliminating, or embedding foods to better meet your child's nutritional needs. For example, one child who was unwilling to eat anything other than chicken nuggets was willing to eat mashed-up veggies formed into the shape of chicken nuggets. You may also learn previously unknown facts about maximizing the vitamin and nutrient benefits of certain foods singularly or in combination.

My child overeats—is there anything I could or should do about it?

Poor eating habits can impact your child's mood and self-image, especially when entering adolescence—a time when he's more likely than ever to feel differently about himself. Your child takes his direction from you, and his eating habits are a learned behavior. What kinds of foods are you purchasing and stocking in your home? What's your policy on fast food, snacking before and after dinner, or prior to bedtime? Can you examine and reassess your own diet in order to create positive changes?

When your child craves sweets, high-fructose caffeinated soft drinks, and carbohydrates loaded with salt, fat, and empty calories, it could be contributing to not only weight gain but irritability and a predisposition to diabetes depending on the degree of sugar intake. Although it's true that genetics may influence a person's weight and body type, some kids with autism are already not as physically coordinated as they may wish to be; this makes regular participation in recreational activities unappealing and without motivation. If you also have a sedentary lifestyle, you are modeling this conduct as acceptable.

In addition to fostering healthier eating habits in consultation with your child's pediatrician and a dietician or nutritionist, you should definitely explore ways in which to introduce a gentle exercise program to your child (see the previous list of suggested activities) in which you may both participate.

I notice that my child's behavior seems to spike after eating certain foods—why is that?

It may depend on precisely *what* your child is consuming. As noted earlier, certain food side effects can create internal warfare for your child's physiology—an experience she may be unable to identify or put language to. Be certain to consult with your child's pediatrician to discuss your concerns and observations. In addition to exploring the gluten- and casein-free diet discussed earlier, some healthy ways to avert such severe reactions may include:

- avoiding foods with artificial dyes and chemical preservatives;
- cutting back on red meat in favor of poultry, seafood, or other protein options;
- serving free-range red meat and poultry, that is, meat and poultry that haven't had antibiotic injections;
- considering soy or other substitute foods;

- reducing or eliminating sugar in sweets, chocolates, cakes, and pastries;
- reducing or eliminating caffeinated soft drinks;
- increasing water intake; and
- introducing more natural fiber from fruits and vegetables.

Such sound dietary measures will benefit your entire family overall if you are able to commit to making gradual adjustments to your menu. Engaging your child with autism to make choices from options you provide, or helping create recipes, will give him reason to feel invested in menu planning and grocery shopping.

My child will urinate appropriately, but how can I get him to move his bowels in the toilet?

Toilet training is a sensitive issue for many children, not just kids on the autism spectrum. There's a difference between standing and confronting the toilet to urinate and submitting to it by turning your back and having your very flesh physically contact it—a daunting prospect for many boys (and for girls who must sit to use the toilet *every* time). There may be any number of reasons why children with autism may have difficulty with the toileting process. Here are a few:

- For some, it may be one of the only ways they can exert any kind of control in their lives if many other aspects of their day—and time spent—are micromanaged.
- Their bodies may not be properly receiving "signals" the brain is sending in time to make it to the toilet.
- Explore a thorough diet review—are there certain foods that are problematic, creating gastrointestinal issues?
- Ever flush a toilet and have it sound like you're going to get sucked down with it because it's got such a roar? Now, magnify that with

the intensity of the child with acute sensory sensitivity for noise, and you've got a terrifying ritual to be avoided at all costs.

- Similarly, for some children, the texture or temperature of the toilet seat may be uncomfortable (and might be remedied by allowing them to select a new model).

- Unless it's been explained to them, some kids on the autism spectrum may panic when moving their bowels, believing that they are shedding a piece of their insides that's not supposed to come out.

- Similarly, some children on the autism spectrum may be in perfectionism mode, and not wish to "get dirty" or become involved in the process of caring for oneself before, during, and after toileting.

- For many young children—especially those with autism—*everything* has the potential to be alive. Is your child certain that the toilet is inanimate?

- Finally, in some children and teens, defecating or smearing feces in places other than the toilet, coupled with the fact that the child ordinarily knows to use the toilet (and has been successful doing so), may point to an emotional or mental health issue that needs to be addressed.

How do I communicate toileting concepts to my child?

The same way in which you'd communicate any important piece of information. For the child who thinks in pictures and movies, you'd convey it visually; for the child who best assimilates auditory information, you'd record and replay it. At the back of this book there's a story written for children with autism struggling with moving their bowels in the toilet, and you may modify it to suit your needs.

For those kids who perceive adults as omnipotent, it's an earth-shattering revelation to realize that everyone they know does this, is supposed to do this, and it's okay to do it! This includes not only family members, but teachers, favorite movie and TV characters—even the president of the United States. (The caution here being that these subjects are discussed privately, not blurted out publicly.) Children who are not well coordinated may need practice reaching around to wipe, "hit" the right spot, and clean themselves without smearing. Automatic-flush toilets have added a new dimension to bathroom anxiety for kids unhinged by the unpredictable, but if you or your child keep a piece of duct tape handy, you can cover the toilet sensor, prevent it from going off unexpectedly, and control when you are ready to allow it to flush. Try going to a hardware store and allowing your child the chance to manipulate a toilet that's not "hooked up" in order to satisfy his curiosity and gain some familiarity and control.

In addition to allaying your child's concerns with these ideas, you may wish to check out the *Once Upon a Potty* books, or an autism spectrum–specific resource like Maria Wheeler's *Toilet Training for Individuals with Autism and Related Disorders*.

I caught my eleven-year-old son pulling on his penis—what should I do about this?

Human beings are sexual beings, and we have all touched ourselves at one time or another. It is natural for children to be curious about their bodies, but when it comes to children and adolescents with different ways of being and their sexuality, we tend not to want to go there because of our own discomfort, a presumption of lesser intellect, or the denial that a child is growing and maturing with sexuality as a facet of their being. Oftentimes, masturbation is one of the few pleasurable ways in which individuals with differences can independently find personal release.

How you approach the matter of masturbation depends on your personal, moral, or religious beliefs about this activity. If you choose to disallow your child's masturbation, please remember that your child most likely retains information about events linked to extreme emotion in a way that is indelible. If you react strongly with great upset, threats, or anger, you have the potential to forever alter your child's perceptions of his body image, his sexuality, and his perception of how others conduct themselves. If you perpetuate old wives' tales about masturbation ("You'll go blind," "You'll grow hair on your palms") in an effort to frighten your child into compliance, he will probably believe what you are telling him as the truth. Be firm yet gentle and sensitive in setting limits.

If you condone masturbation as normal and natural, you'll want to instill in your child the concept of "public" versus "private" conduct. You'll also want to ensure that your child is not going to harm himself by being too rough. A direct and graphic story explaining masturbation for males is located at the back of this book; it may be revised to meet the needs of females. In addition, there have been a burgeoning number of recent books addressing the puberty and sexuality needs of young people with autism.

How do I help my daughter with autism understand menstruation?

Communicating the sequence of this physical transformation and its personal hygiene care for females with autism is a task of prevention. Recall the child who is unnerved by a small paper cut because it's visible and excretes blood? Menstruation is also a very visual process, and it will be important to explain to your daughter as calmly and as gently as possible that menstruation is a *natural* process and one that is not intended to create fear or panic.

As with all important matters, this concept will need to be conveyed as simply and as visually as possible, and as often as is needed, to provide your daughter with the assurances and comfort level she'll require to make peace with this new change within her. Basic information such as premenstrual symptoms, ways to gain relief for pain and discomfort, and the idea of a "clean pad" versus a "red pad" should be incorporated into this discussion. One Internet resource that provides a sample story with some picture icons may offer you a starting point for gathering ideas. It can be found, in two parts, at

http://members.cox.net/tinsnips/Media/menstruation1.pdf and http://members.cox.net/tinsnips/Media/menstruation2.pdf.

Chapter 6

MENTAL HEALTH

- What is causing my child to have so much trouble sleeping?
- What kind of medication should be prescribed for my child's inability to sleep?
- Are there natural alternatives to medication as a sleep aid?
- Is being anxious all the time associated with being having autism?
- Aren't my child's aggressive "acting-out" behaviors simply a part of autism?
- How do I manage my child's angry outbursts and frustration?
- Could acting out or misbehaving be a sign that a child's emotional needs are not being met?
- Is my child with autism more likely to suffer from depression than other children?
- What are the signs of depression that parents should be aware of?
- What medications for depression are most often used with children with good success and few side effects?
- What if the problem is not depression?
- What is bipolar disorder?
- What is oppositional defiant disorder?
- What is intermittent explosive disorder?
- What are the alternatives to psychotropic drugs that are currently being promoted by some doctors and drug companies to control extreme autistic behaviors?
- Are medication supplements effective?
- How do I find a doctor qualified to attend to my child's mental health needs?
- What should I be looking for when seeking a doctor to help in the mental health treatment of my child?
- How long will it take to get my child a mental health diagnosis?
- Are my child's mental health experiences my fault?
- Is my child more likely to experience post-traumatic stress disorder when something bad happens to him?
- How will I know if my child has PTSD?
- How do I keep my child safe during a meltdown?
- How do I stay safe if my child is having a meltdown?
- Do I need to hospitalize my child for mental health issues?
- Can my child's mental health be stabilized?

What is causing my child to have so much trouble sleeping?

The quality of your child's sleep has a direct impact on her ability to be productive and to function optimally. Difficulty sleeping or sleep disturbances are common among young children on the autism spectrum, and may often be traced to emotional or anxiety-related issues. There may be several reasons why your child is having a hard time shutting down to sleep at night.

First, never underestimate the exquisite sensitivity your child may experience. Could her inability to sleep be attributed to too much or too little light in the room, or too much or too little noise? Some people prefer to fall asleep to a television or radio, or will play a soothing relaxation CD to help them drift off—might this be of use for your child?

Is your child sensitive to tension or strong emotions occurring in the house? If you trace the beginnings of your child's sleep difficulties, do they coincide with stressful circumstances that you thought your child couldn't sense or overhear? You may be surprised at the ways in which many young children, autistic or not, perceive adults' vibes. Or is your child magnifying fears brought on by something seen or heard on TV?

Finally, many children with autism also experience acute anxiety brought on by their dependency on adults for information about what's coming next. Developing a visual list or schedule with your child for the following day and going over it just prior to bedtime should help immeasurably.

What kind of medication should be prescribed for my child's inability to sleep?

A number of medications can be used short term to provide your child (and you) some relief from restless or sleepless nights.

However, if you decide to explore this option, please know that medication is just one piece of a solution. Up to 80 percent of prescription medications have not been FDA approved for use in children and were tested only on adults. The appropriate dosage will be determined by your child's pediatrician. Some medications that have been prescribed for children for their effectiveness include:

- Ambien;
- Sonata;
- benzodiazepines like Ativan, Valium, Librium, Xanax, Halcion, and ProSom;
- melatonin;
- Benadryl;
- clonidine; and
- Tenex.

All medications come with side effects that will require careful monitoring and close consultation with the doctor. If you believe your child has a medication-related emergency and your doctor is unavailable, contact the Poison Control Center at 1-800-222-1222.

Are there natural alternatives to medication as a sleep aid?

Parents who are wary of introducing medication into their child's system may wish to pursue homeopathic remedies that contain common, natural botanical ingredients in order to avert medication side effects such as addiction, grogginess, nightmares, or increased insomnia. Ask your child's pediatrician about homeopathic alternatives to medication, or consult your telephone directory for a homeopathic practitioner near you. Your local holistic or all-natural food center may be a resource for learning more about supplements that may induce a relaxed state in your child in order to promote sleep. If your child is allergy sensitive, be particularly mindful of avoiding natural alternatives that contain the ingredient to which she is allergic. Some of the popular homeopathic sleep aids include Herbal Rest, Sleep Aid Herbal Formula, DuDu Kiddie Sleep Remedy, and Serenite Jr.

Other options include warm baths scented with pleasant-smelling bath oil, listening to soft, relaxing music, reading a story, or talking about the day's events right before bedtime. One mom has a tip that has helped her son: "A friend of mine showed me a small flannel bag filled with rice and lavender flowers. You place it in the microwave to heat it, and then give it to your child so he can go to sleep with it. The lavender is relaxing, and the warmth of the rice is soothing."

Is being anxious all the time associated with having autism?

Not necessarily, although many children on the autism spectrum deal with anxiety issues. Usually, the anxiety, which may manifest in irritability, clinginess, trouble sleeping, and extremely rigid behavior, may be traced to feeling out of control. Too often, adults and care-givers seem to be the keepers of so much information that does not get shared about what's coming next. For the child already besieged by difficulties processing information about his world, there may be an innate need to exert control through rigid adherence to routines and schedules in order to offset worrisome or consuming thoughts about not knowing what to expect. So much anxiety could be quelled (and medication discontinued) if we simply disciplined ourselves to presume the intellect of our children and carefully and thoroughly explained what's coming next far enough in advance to give the child with autism time to plan and prepare.

Aren't my child's aggressive "acting-out" behaviors simply a part of autism?

It is a myth and stereotype that verbally and physically aggressive behavior is directly associated with autism. If you are presuming your child's intellect, you will appreciate that he has good reasons for doing what he's doing, and understand that he's doing the very best that he knows how to in the moment—wouldn't you justify your own actions and behavior in the same way?

Given this principle, you may wish to revisit any demonstration of your child's aggressive actions—especially if he does not talk—in terms of *communication*, not behavior. It may be that your child's "behaviors" can be attributed to one, or a combination of, the following:

- the inability to communicate (speak) in ways that are effective, reliable, and universally understandable;
- the inability to communicate his own physical pain and discomfort (including sensory sensitivities) in ways that are effective, reliable, and universally understandable; and
- the inability to communicate his own mental health experience (including emotional pain and distress) in ways that are effective, reliable, and universally understandable.

Working from the premise of deciphering the source of your child's aggression in this manner may assist you in processing his outbursts from an objective, not subjective, point of view, by perceiving his actions as *reactions*.

How do I manage my child's angry outbursts and frustration?

First, consider the household tone you set for what is acceptable behavior. If you are short tempered and quick to anger, you are modeling this behavior as acceptable. Your home should be your child's safe haven, free from the emotional and environmental stressors she is combating throughout the day. Does your home offer a private space for your child to play or decompress, or is it chaotic?

Your child with autism may view the world as scrambled, fragmented, and disconnected. It is understandable that your child's very sensitive tolerance level would regularly "max out," and one way she may attempt to gain control is through angry and rigid insistence, especially when it comes to a requirement for sameness. In what manner can you offer your child some measure of control and the luxury of making choices on a daily basis? This may decrease your child's need to assert control through angry outbursts.

Part of parenting your child with autism means also fostering the development of self-advocacy. One mom tells of working toward this process with her daughter: "She doesn't understand after a major tantrum (at age twelve) why everyone around her is still upset once it's over. We've been working a lot on self-control and self-awareness. She can't handle the amount of words spoken to her, and hates talking about 'issues.' We have started to write letters to her, because she can accept that more easily." One published resource designed to help kids on the autism spectrum gain the upper hand is *When My Autism Gets Too Big! A Relaxation Book for Children with Autism Spectrum Disorders* by Kari Dunn Buron and Brenda Myles Smith.

Could acting out or misbehaving be a sign that a child's emotional needs are not being met?

That may be one way to interpret what's going on; and if you're a parent suggesting it as a possibility, it stands to reason there may be some truth to it. Raising any child is a joyful, unpredictable, and stressful experience; raising a child with significant differences from what's considered "the norm" can magnify (or overwhelm) your parenting responsibilities.

It is no secret that there is a high divorce rate among parents of children with disabilities. How you and your spouse, or the significant other in your life, choose to cope with your stress can impact your child, his emotional well-being, and his perception of his place in the family. If you're a "Type A" personality—someone who is driven or distracted by lots of priorities—parenting a child with autism may require you to slow down and assess how you manage your time in order to meet the emotional needs of all your children, but especially your child with autism, who may be predisposed to feeling insecure and anxious.

Is my child with autism more likely to suffer from depression than other children?

As someone who is inherently gentle and exquisitely sensitive, and as someone who must daily yield to an unpredictable and intolerant world, your child is more likely to grapple with depression. This potential is compounded if you, your spouse, or an immediate or extended family member is also depressed or is dealing with another significant mental health experience. It means that heredity may influence your child's vulnerability to a depressed state.

Genetics aside, *anyone* who has trouble communicating, sustaining social connections, and expressing pain or sensory sensitivities and who doesn't consistently have his or her intellect presumed would become depressed! If you've ever experienced a prolonged and debilitating condition, such as speech or mobility loss, you may be able to better empathize with such feelings of hopelessness and low self-esteem. Your child is likely to first begin showing signs of depression on the precipice of adolescence—a time when she may develop a heightened awareness of her differences or may be ostracized by her peers because of them.

What are the signs of depression that parents should be aware of?

Watch for changes in behavior that are unusual or noticeably different from what is typical for your child, especially spikes of irritability, complaints, and melancholy. Is there a decreased interest or indifference for things your child previously enjoyed doing? Also monitor for changes in sleep patterns (up at all hours of the night, or difficulty rousing your child in the morning), eating habits (hoarding or bingeing on sweets or carbs, or reduced appetite), and a general apathy, inability to concentrate, or inability to complete an activity within regular time frames.

If your child seems preoccupied with morbid topics such as warfare, disease, accidents, cemeteries, death and dying, or if your child is making self-deprecating remarks about being unloved or desiring to hurt themselves (or is doing so through self-injury), take immediate action; do not wait to see if this will pass. Childhood depression is a serious matter, and you will wish to consult with your child's pediatrician promptly to report your concerns in terms of symptoms—not behaviors.

What medications for depression are most often used with children with good success and few side effects?

When it comes to treating mental health issues in anyone, there are no rules. That is, although mental illness is an equal opportunity offender, it affects each individual uniquely; no clinician can state with certainty that what successfully works for one person will work for another. Finding a proper plan of support is a process—an often frustrating one—that can be time consuming.

As discussed for sleep aid medications, antidepressant medications have not been FDA approved for use in persons under age eighteen;

so should your child's doctor prescribe such medication, she is doing so at her professional discretion using her clinical best judgment. In fact, the FDA mandates that antidepressant medications must bear a warning label indicating the increased risk of suicidal thinking and behavior in children and adolescents.

Any success with an antidepressant may vary significantly depending on your child's age, metabolism, severity of depression, and unique physiology. In addition to treating depression, antidepressant medication may be prescribed for anxiety, panic attacks, phobias, eating disorders, and attention deficit/hyperactivity disorder (ADHD). Consult with your child's doctor, research online, and ask questions of your local pharmacist regarding any information you require to learn more about antidepressant medication and its benefits and side effects.

What if the problem is not depression?

If you have researched the symptoms of depression and you believe your child is likely depressed, but her doctor has ruled out depression, you may wish to consider seeking a second opinion. Remember, there is still a prevailing belief among some clinicians that any "noncompliant behavior" in someone with a developmental disability is simply an expected by-product of that person's condition.

If your child's doctor has ruled out depression, was another diagnosis such as anxiety disorder or post-traumatic stress disorder made instead? It is possible that your child's symptoms are a better "fit" with a mental health experience other than depression.

Yet, due to its commonality in us all, depression should be thoroughly explored while examining other possibilities; the *Diagnostic and Statistical Manual of Mental Disorders* recommends this approach by advising the consideration of mood disorders foremost, which includes depression.

If your child's doctor has not made a diagnosis, ask for her professional recommendations for supporting your child's changing mood through alternatives modes and techniques including proper diet, rest and exercise combined with making compassionate accommodations for your child's unique sensory and emotional requirements. Trust your parental instincts and remain firm in advocating the needs of your child with autism.

What is bipolar disorder?

Bipolar disorder is clinically classified as a mood disorder, and comprises two extreme mood variations: depression and mania. (At one time, persons with bipolar disorder were disrespectfully referred to as "manic-depressives.") If you break it down, *bi* means two, so *bipolar* pertains to two opposite poles, or two extremes. No one can tell when or how often someone's mood will fluctuate; it may be months or minutes—again, there are no rules. There is a growing belief among psychiatrists and psychologists that children with bipolar disorder may, in fact, be misdiagnosed with ADHD instead.

As is true of depression, being bipolar is no one's fault and may be attributed to any combination of factors such as family history or abuse and trauma. In the case of the child with autism, being exquisitely sensitive and without a means to communicate chronic frustration and pain—let alone wants, needs, and desires—may predispose your child to a mental health experience. Bipolar disorder is among the most common mental health diagnoses in the typical population, and yet persons with autism are often misdiagnosed, or their symptoms are perceived as autistic "behaviors" and go untreated.

In the child with autism, the manic portion of bipolar disorder will most likely grab attention for its intensity. Watch for *euphoric mood*, which is a distinct increase in silliness, teasing, laughing (sometimes a different-sounding laugh), irritability, and excessive grinning. Also monitor for *grandiosity* (a sense of inflated self-esteem and impor-tance); you'll see this if your child becomes very bossy, tells you she's in charge, pushes or physically manipulates others, and/or destroys property (especially with lots of unusual strength). Children who are grandiose may refer to themselves as movie or cartoon characters, and may even disregard using the toilet as they had been. Other signs of possible manic mood include the need for very little sleep, if any at all; increased appetite; constantly moving beyond what's typical; high distractibility; talking or vocalizing hard and fast; and jumping from topic to topic with no correlation (or, in the nonspeaking child, moving from place to place with no agenda).

On the Internet, you may wish to check out any number of websites for kids who are bipolar, including www.bpchildren.com, www.bpkids.net, and www.bipolarchild.com.

What is oppositional defiant disorder?

Oppositional defiant disorder (ODD) is a clinical diagnosis with symptoms that can mimic those of bipolar disorder. ODD manifests in a hostile, persistent trend of behaviors that could easily be misin-terpreted as defiance, stubbornness, ballistic temper, and defying authority figures (i.e., you!). Its symptoms occur more often in younger boys than girls, but affect both sexes equally after puberty.

To be considered for an ODD diagnosis, you should observe four or more of the following behaviors in your child for the past six months or more:

- Loses temper.
- Argues with adults.
- Refuses to follow rules or conform to adult requests.
- Deliberately does things to agitate others.
- Blames others for bad behavior or for accidents or mistakes.

- Displays overall mood of anger and resentment.
- Exhibits vengeful or spiteful behavior.

Do your best to avoid categorizing your child's aggressive actions as merely symptoms of her autistic experience; remember, she is likely communicating her dissatisfaction or frustration in the only way she knows how. As always, when in doubt, consult with your child's pediatrician, or request a referral to a pediatric psychiatrist.

What is intermittent explosive disorder?

Intermittent explosive disorder (IED) is another mental health diagnosis that is a collection of violent, out-of-control, and unpredictable behaviors known as impulse-control disorders. IED is the inability to resist aggressive impulses to cause destruction and harm to others (in males this can include sexual acting out). Although it is generally diagnosed in persons past adolescence, it has also been applied to children with developmental disabilities, children with ADHD, and children with other types of conduct concerns.

To qualify for IED, other diagnoses, including the possibility of a manic episode, are to be ruled out first, and the rage manifested must be out of proportion to the type and degree of stressor that precedes such an episode. Many clinicians feel that IED is reflective of traits of another mental health diagnosis; and, indeed, it shares elements of bipolar symptoms such as spikes in irritability, racing thoughts, and intensified energy that escalates in an explosive outburst, after which a depressed mood may arise.

IED is considered uncommon and generally appears in males. Please consult with your child's pediatrician for further information about intermittent explosive disorder or any other mental health experiences. It is proper to consider ongoing severe mood changes as an issue adjunct to your child's autism, but it is equally important to be careful and methodical in gathering information that may lead to an accurate mental health diagnosis.

What are the alternatives to psychotropic drugs that are currently being promoted by some doctors and drug companies to control extreme autistic behaviors?

These days you can't turn on the television without seeing advertisements for medication of one kind or another, and it may seem as though a concerted campaign has been mounted to promote drugs as "quick fixes." That shouldn't deter you from considering the benefit and value of medication as *part of* an overall plan of wellness for your child, a plan that should also take into account nutrition and exercise.

If you have reservations about psychotropic medications (medications used to contain and control psychotic derangement), it may be because you are fearful of strong side effects, your child does not respond well to medication or is allergic, or you are uncomfortable with a proposed plan of treatment. Alternatives to medication may be an option you will wish to explore. Among the natural supplements to consider are:

- 5-HTP, an amino acid extract that has been shown to be helpful in treating depression and bipolarity;
- omega-3, a polyunsaturated fatty acid found in fish oil, flaxseed, pumpkin seed, and walnuts, that has been shown to aid in balancing symptoms of ADHD, depression, and bipolarity;
- St. John's wort, an herb derivative used to treat anxiety, depression, and sleeplessness;
- Sam-e, a natural compound that works with the body's folic acid and vitamin B-12 to reduce symptoms of depression; and
- B vitamins, a deficiency of which can mimic or exacerbate bipolar symptoms.

To learn more about these supplements, check online or with your local holistic health center, but always consult with your child's pediatrician prior to introducing your child to any supplement, singularly or in combination.

Are medication supplements effective?

As with any new treatment method, this depends entirely on your child and her physiology, lifestyle, and support system. Just because a medication supplement is a natural alternative doesn't mean it is harmless for children, that more is better, or that it is without side effects or possible interactions with other conditions. (Be mindful, too, that holistic health practitioners who treat their clients with unconventional methods are not subject to regulated standards in the way that traditional physicians are.)

Before considering the effectiveness of a medication or natural supplement, be aware that many of them, including those previously listed, should not be taken in conjunction with medication used to treat depression or bipolar disorder. Information about their effectiveness in children is not well documented, so any dosage determination would need to be highly individualized and monitored closely. Natural supplements may be an attractive and viable alternative to aid in stabilizing your child's mood, and there are kids who do benefit from them, but there is no certainty as to their efficacy in your child without consulting closely with your doctor.

How do I find a doctor qualified to attend to my child's mental health needs?

The best place to begin your search for a clinician qualified to treat your child's mental health needs is to ask your child's pediatrician. Your child's doctor may not be in a position to make a mental health diagnosis, but she may have a general working knowledge of what to look for as out of the ordinary behavior. As such, she may be an excellent resource in giving you advice about what to be further exploring, and may be able to make a referral to a colleague, or will know of a reputable pediatric psychologist or psychiatrist.

In addition, you could try the child psychiatry department of the local university or hospital, or you may find a doctor through contacts made from connections with other parents of kids with autism. You may also wish to use the search engine on the website of the American Academy of Child and Adolescent Psychiatry (www.acap.org) to locate any number of qualified doctors in your state who may be a resource to you and your child.

What should I be looking for when seeking a doctor to help in the mental health treatment of my child?

If you live in a rural area, you may be tempted to pursue the clinician who is closest to you; in a metropolitan area, you may have your pick of professionals without feeling the need to be particularly choosy. In either instance, do not be swayed by convenience. Instead, you will wish to consider any or all of the following:

- Does the doctor come highly recommended?
- Does the doctor treat all kids, including those with developmental differences?
- Does the doctor have experience in distinguishing autism from mental health issues?
- Does the doctor keep current with trends in autism, or does the doctor cling to old schools of thought?
- Does the doctor seem to be a good listener, someone with whom you will feel comfortable partnering?
- Does the doctor accept your insurance?
- Does the doctor have a good rapport with your child or did the

doctor attempt to diagnose him from across the room?
- Does your child like the doctor?

Finding a clinician to support your child's mental health needs may be a process of trial and error until you find someone with whom you feel trustworthy and who seems committed to working with you and your child. Be prepared not to find this professional down the block, but quite possibly in a neighboring county, across the state, in a large medical center, or across state lines.

How long will it take to get my child a mental health diagnosis?

Determining a mental health diagnosis *and* matching the diagnosis with adequate and appropriate clinical treatment is a process that can take years for anyone in need of treatment, let alone the child with autism and a mental health experience. A good mental health clinician would confide that all of psychiatry is guesswork, albeit educated guesswork; but, because it is not an exacting science, it truly does boil down to respectful speculation.

Once you locate a child psychiatrist or psychologist, that person should spend time interviewing you and your child, listen carefully to your concerns, observe your child closely, and be available to answer any questions you may have. Understand that your mental health clinician is well educated and is in the business of helping you and your child, but also know that individual is extremely vulnerable to whatever information you share (i.e., if you vent about aggressive, out-of-control "behaviors" versus discussing possible symptoms), in addition to the manner, tone, and context in which you share it.

You can minimize the guesswork on the part of your child's mental health practitioner by communicating as concisely and as nonemotionally as possible; cooperating when asked questions without being defensive, evasive, or protective by withholding information; and being clear in discussing symptoms, not behaviors. When you do this, the doctor is better poised to develop a clearer snapshot of your child's experience to help lead to an accurate diagnosis.

Are my child's mental health experiences my fault?

If you are sensitive enough to ask if your child's mental health experiences could be attributed to something you've caused, then you are most likely the type of parent who is loving, caring, considerate, and doing everything within your power to support your child. Mental health experiences can, though, be induced as a by-product of unloving, abusive parent–child relationships, as we've read about or heard about in the media. In extreme instances, apart from or inclusive of other forms of abuse, a parent (usually a mother) will intentionally create a hostile environment in order to perpetuate or prolong a child's developmental, physical, or mental health experience because it brings that parent attention and sympathy from the family, the community, and prevailing professionals. These circumstances do not directly pertain to autism exclusively.

As you've learned, genetics has been considered as a leading possibility for influencing autism; but if you, your spouse, or a family member on either side has a history of mental health experiences this can impact your child with autism as well. It does not mean you are at fault in any way; do not berate yourself for something outside of your control. It simply means that your child may be extra sensitive and predisposed to the same or similar mental health issues.

Is my child more likely to experience post-traumatic stress disorder when something bad happens to him?

Bad is a relative and subjective term, one that, in this instance, can be determined only by your child. As a person with autism, your child is naturally and inherently gentle and exquisitely sensitive. What this means in terms of teasing, scolding, and name-calling is that he cannot necessarily "buck up," "snap out of it," or "get over it" in the way that you might or your other children can. Many people with autism, especially those who think in pictures, retain and replay unpleasant and hurtful experiences, and this can impede one's mental health.

Children who have participated in, been the recipient of, or have observed abuse of any kind or witnessed a violent event like a natural catastrophe or accident are at tremendous risk of developing a condition know as post-traumatic stress disorder (PTSD). PTSD is defined by symptoms that usually manifest within three months of the event, but in a child with autism the aftereffects may be immediate. Depression is also a mental health experience often occurring simultaneously with PTSD.

How will I know if my child has PTSD?

Consult your child's pediatrician in a timely manner if any of the following symptoms are manifesting in a way that significantly impairs the quality of your child's life:

- Seems overly fearful or clingy.
- Appears to reenact an abusive act or attempts to perpetrate it on another.
- Has nightmares, night terrors, and night sweats.
- Seems "hypervigilant"; is always on guard and unable to relax.

- Is even more withdrawn socially than usual.
- Starts wetting the bed.
- Is communicating the experience through art, music, writing, or poetry.
- Has outbursts of irritability.
- Feels unsafe in familiar environments.
- Is fearful of someone who was previously trusted.
- "Zones out" or seems to have flashbacks triggered by a sensory experience that relates to the traumatizing event.

The child with autism who does not speak may be at greater risk of PTSD resulting from abuse because he is a silent witness and a silent victim, especially if a perpetrator does not presume intellect.

How do I keep my child safe during a meltdown?

Even if you've been diligent in applying the principle of "prevention instead of intervention" as it pertains to the environments in which your child may find himself, there will always be those unanticipated circumstances over which you have no control that will arise to unhinge him. If your child is unable to communicate his symptoms of escalating anxiety, and gives you no warning signs, he may lose control in a very obvious and public manner. You can employ a number of strategies to minimize the severity of the situation and protect your child's safety:

- Remain as calm as possible. It won't help if your mood, despair, or temper flares in correlation with that of your child.
- Speak to your child by name in a low, even, and nonemotional tone of voice.
- Speak clearly, directly, and concisely, using as few words as possible in order to direct your child to a safe escape from the

situation (i.e., "Tyler, this way please").

- Pair your words with visuals such as pointing or motioning to the place where you'd like your child to go with you.
- Repeat the same exact phrases over again as needed.
- Acknowledge what is happening and offer your assurances that it will be okay.
- Gently guide your child with a touch at the shoulder, arm, or elbow and begin moving with him.
- If all else fails, try to talk your child into sitting on the floor with you hugging him from behind and consciously deep breathing to de-escalate.

Once your child is able to regain control, and you are both in a safe and quiet place, you may wish to process what just happened in order to glean information from your child (if he's able to communicate it) about what triggered his reaction; you may be surprised by the one detail in the environment you overlooked.

How do I stay safe when my child is having a meltdown?

Children grow quickly, and your young child with autism and potential mental health issues won't stay small forever. In fact, as he grows it may become more and more difficult to deal with the intensity of outbursts or physical aggression, and to protect your child—and yourself and your family. If you are concurrently seeking mental health treatment and know your child has the potential to do physical harm in the form of hitting, scratching, pulling hair, or using objects as weapons, you may want to look into a safety techniques training program offered at your local community center, human services agency provider, or hospital. During quiet times, be clear and firm (using visuals) about what is acceptable and not acceptable behavior.

Also in the spirit of preventive measures, you may consider any of the following tips:

- Disallow any overtly violent or sexually graphic music, movies, videos, and computer games in your home.
- Install locks high enough for only you to reach or, if feasible, an alarm system on your doors and windows.
- Remove or replace all hanging glass picture frames.
- Lock up guns, knives, scissors, razors, fireplace pokers, sports equipment, and work tools that could become a spontaneous weapon.
- Keep expensive, large appliances (TVs, computers) in a locked room to avoid destruction.
- Be mindful of the needs of pets, siblings, and other family members during such incidents.

Many potentially tragic circumstances can be avoided through these and other methods of prevention.

Do I need to hospitalize my child for mental health issues?

Hospitalization can be a scary prospect for both you and your child; but in times of overwhelming duress, you may feel as if it is your only option. You may reach such a point if you find yourself regularly attempting to keep your child, yourself, and your family safe from harm. Do not wait until circumstances reach total crisis in order to explore the details for short-term hospitalization with your child's doctor; gather as much information as possible in order to make an informed choice *before* things escalate out of control. The last thing you want is for your child to be forcibly taken away in an ambulance or—worse yet—a police car.

The determination to commit a child to psychiatric hospitalization is usually made if he or she is a danger to themselves or others.

That is, if the health, safety, and welfare of your family is at stake, or if your child has seriously injured himself, there's been no improvement, and you can no longer guarantee his safety at home, school, or the community.

Most large hospitals have a children's psychiatric ward that you may wish to inquire about to learn how much the staff know about kids with autism (you'll want to be present with your child as much as possible), what kinds of physical restraints might be used, what kinds of medications might be administered and for what purpose, and what a typical stay is like. The goal of any psychiatric hospitalization is safe and efficient stabilization of your child's mental health before discharge.

Can my child's mental health be stabilized?

The stabilization of anyone's mental health is a process; stabilizing the mental heath needs of the child with autism can be challenged by the difficulty of separating mental health symptoms from autistic symptoms, accurately tracking and reporting data such as cycles or trends, and your child's inability to communicate her own mental health experience. The truth is that it may be a frustrating trial-and-error process that will put your parenting skills and parental love to task. If your child's mental health requires stabilization, she is depending on you to advocate her needs for her, to never give up, and to hold true to hope and optimism. The world is shifting—albeit slowly—toward a greater awareness of autism; and your role, in partnership with your child, can be that of a teacher to support that change in positive ways.

Chapter 7

VALUING PASSIONS

- What is a *passion*?
- Isn't *stimming*, I mean, *self-soothing*, a passion?
- What is meant by "valuing" passions?
- What do I do when I've been told the opposite—that I need to stop my child's passion?
- How do I determine my child's passion?
- Can my child have more than one passion?
- Can my child's passion change over time?
- What if my child doesn't have a passion?
- Does my child's diagnosis of obsessive-compulsive disorder refer to his passion or something else?
- Is it possible for my child's passion to turn into OCD?
- Should I allow my child to be involved in her passion as much as she wants?
- My son's passion is the computer and video games—should I limit him to two hours a day?
- How come my child doesn't want to share his passion with me, only with strangers?
- Should I use my child's passion as a reward to be earned?
- Should I punish my child by withholding his passion?
- What do I do if, in the past, I have punished my child by withholding her passion?
- Is it okay for my child to have lots of "online friends" and play lots of online games?
- How do I respond when my child's teacher says his need to talk about his passion is disruptive?
- How do I handle it when my child's passion seems to be isolating him socially because it is no longer appropriate for his age?
- Can my child's passion be used as a learning tool?
- Is it possible for my child's passion to become her job one day?
- Will my child's passion hinder him from developing romantic relationships some day?
- How do I help others to see the value of my child's passion when they often see it as a nuisance or OCD?
- Is my child gifted in his passion?
- What can I do to further encourage my child's passion?

What is a *passion*?

The topic or subject area in which your child with autism is absolutely and enjoyably absorbed is his passion. Given his druthers, he would spend all his free time reading about, drawing, talking about, watching on television, researching on the Internet, or reenacting this topic. You may also hear passions referred to as "special interests." Some examples of areas of passion for any number of kids with autism include, but are not limited to, the following:

- cartoon characters and animation;
- computer games;
- dinosaurs;
- oceanography;
- astronomy;
- trains or anything with wheels;
- music of all kinds but particularly classical;
- U.S. presidents;
- specific films such as *Harry Potter*, *Star Wars*, *Star Trek*, or *The Wizard of Oz*; or
- famous scientists, researchers, or celebrities.

Isn't *stimming,* I mean *self-soothing,* a passion?

No. Self-soothing or self-regulating actions or activities such as repetitively twirling a piece of string, flapping one's hands, or perpetual rocking do not qualify as passions. These actions are intended to maintain a sense of order, safety, and control. You may, though, see your child using time indulged in her passion similarly to the way she uses a self-soothing or self-regulating action or activity; that is, your child may engage in her passion to decompress and reorganize and may appear oblivious to all else during these times. However, a calming action or vocalization is not the same thing as a passion for a topic or subject matter.

Nor do food and eating count as a passion *unless* your child is endlessly fascinated by cooking shows, loves to help cook, operates kitchen appliances, creates new recipes, follows the careers of celebrity chefs, and loves to shop for food. Otherwise, your child's intense desire to consume food may simply be a reflection of something pleasurable that involves all the senses and which he may look forward to on a daily basis.

What is meant by "valuing" passions?

Valuing passions means that you don't misinterpret (or be led by others to misinterpret) your child's strong interest as a behavioral symptom of autism, one that should be extinguished. You must remain firm on this. Instead, perceive your child's passion as having purpose as an expression of dedication and creativity. It is a communication of your child's strengths, gifts, and talents, and should be viewed as an opportunity to make a connection in the context of building a relationship.

What do I do when I've been told the opposite—that I need to stop my child's passion?

How come the people telling you to squelch your child's passion can have a hobby, but define your child's special interest as a pathology? You may, in fact, wish to challenge those very persons by proposing this paradox. However well intentioned they may be, their mind-set stems from PDD clinical criteria that label these devoted interests or activities as pathological; several popular theories call for them to be restricted or eliminated. Your child's passion is thus perceived as abnormal, something that must be stopped in order to "normalize" your child. Your child's very identity is likely to be closely aligned with her most passionate of interests, and it may be extremely upsetting if anyone tries to take it away for good. Read on for further discussion about this special alignment.

How do I determine my child's passion?

If your child with autism communicates fluently, his passion should already be well known to you because it's the one thing you hear him talking about nonstop with great ardor. You've likely been the recipient of dissertation-length explanations of the minute nuances and trivia of whatever it is he takes greatest pleasure in. You may have been given pop quizzes on facets of a topic your child feels you should have fully absorbed by now. Or maybe you notice your child spending lots of free time building, drawing, and designing elaborate and detailed representations of his creative outlet. You may be stunned by the quality and complexity with which your child renders his fascination.

If your child with autism does not speak, pay very careful attention to her eye contact, body language, and facial expressions—this will guide you in making respectful best guesses as to what may relate to her passion. Common areas of strong interest for people with autism who live in silence often include:

- nature—trees, flowers, rivers, ponds, and streams;
- animals (and observing them) of all kinds, from whales to butterflies;
- music—specific genres and musical artists;
- religion and spirituality; and
- relationships with family, especially grandparents.

As you begin to accrue information about a passion for your child who doesn't speak, you will notice the distinct way in which her passion causes her to absolutely light up, become excited and engaged, smile and laugh with great joy, or become enraptured—

able to sit still and attend longer than any other time. These kinds of glowing reactions will aid you in garnering more information about the topic areas your child seems most drawn to in order to cultivate her interest further.

Can my child have more than one passion?

Your child can absolutely have more than one passion, although you are probably most keenly aware of his foremost passion. Just as may be true of anyone else, there is no limit to the number of topics for which your child may demonstrate aptitude. You may, though, notice patterns or trends that link your child's primary passion with his "subpassions." For example, the child who loves oceanography may be knowledgeable about animal rights activism or how global warming is impacting sea life. The child who loves computers may have an affinity for high-profile software designers or the geography and culture of the locations at which certain computers are manufactured. Another child who loves Greek and Roman mythology may be intrigued by ancient architecture or the renowned philosophers of that period in history. Of course, this does not mean that, as a child with autism, your child is *required* to have more than one passion; it may very well be that your child's primary passion is expansive enough to hold his attention and keep him happily preoccupied just as it is.

Can my child's passion change over time?

Your interests have certainly changed since you were a youngster, and the same may hold true of your child—remember, we are all more alike than we are different, and your child's personal interests may gain momentum or dwindle and fade as he grows and matures, is exposed to new learning opportunities, becomes inspired by indulgent educators or a kind acquaintance, and experiences more of the big world.

You may see your child retain steadfast dedication to his primary passion throughout his childhood, adolescence, and young adulthood. Or your child may lose interest in one area of passion and transition away from it as he develops interest in another area. Either way, you will want to keep current with whatever your child is most passionate about at the moment in order to connect, initiate dialogue, monitor how he spends his time, and strengthen your parent–child relationship by demonstrating your interest in learning all about your child's passion.

What if my child doesn't have a passion?

Your child does indeed have a passion; it's just concealed from you—purposefully or not. If your child's passion is deliberately concealed from you, it is probably because you or another person in his life have misinterpreted it as a purposeless trait of autism that should be suppressed. If you haven't been presuming of intellect and you've worked to extinguish your child's passion, you may well have succeeded. But your child may have a *natural* proclivity for a gift or talent or area of special interest simply by being who he is, and if you've expressed consternation, exasperation, or intolerance for your child's passion and he develops a new one, you can bet you will be the last to know about it.

If you are unaware of your child's passion due to happenstance, it may be because you are not looking hard enough. Have you carefully considered the tips for discerning the passion of a child who is not as communicative as she would want to be? Additionally, when you presume intellect, you'll be better poised to rightfully interpret the oftentimes *symbolic* connotations of a passion that seems age inappropriate. Remember, you determine what your child knows of the world by what you choose to expose her to. Is it really still an interest in *Barney* at age eleven, or is it a burgeoning interest in dinosaurs, better understanding relationships, or teaching? Is it playing with Matchbox cars, or is it a desire to learn more about mechanics that propel a vehicle to race? By paying attention and taking the initiative to offer your child learning opportunities beyond what's on the surface, you may successfully and fully help develop your child's passion.

Does my child's diagnosis of obsessive-compulsive disorder refer to his passion or something else?

Your child's diagnosis of obsessive-compulsive disorder (OCD) may pertain to both his passion *and* his self-soothing or self-regulating action or activity. It really depends on what you've observed, the context in which you've observed it (is the passion being used to decompress?), how you've reported this information to a diagnosing clinician, and whether you see any value to your child's passion. Your child's educators and other professionals may not be in a place where they yet understand the importance of valuing passions, so that they may be coloring your impressions by reporting "OCD behaviors" or "fixations" improperly.

Remember, any clinician—especially one not current with the newest trends in autism—is vulnerable to whatever information you share; your child being diagnosed as having OCD can largely depend on the tone you set and how you frame what your child experiences when you describe it to the clinician. Are you able to distinguish a passion from a self-soothing technique? If so, is it urgent or worrisome enough to even seek a diagnosis? Read on to the next two questions and their responses—they may provide further clarity on this issue.

Is it possible for my child's passion to turn into OCD?

Any regular activity has the potential to become an all-consuming ritual for anyone affected by OCD. OCD in your child with autism may be brought on by stress, anxiety, feelings of inadequacy, or as an adjunct to other mental health experiences. As important as it is not to label your child's passion as an obsession, a passion may become true OCD if its intensity crosses a line, seeps over it, and begins to significantly impair your child's quality of everyday life. Warning signs may prevail if your child's desire to engage in his passion:

- is keeping him awake at night;
- is preoccupying his time so much that he is not hungry or rushes through meals;
- seems to be increasing his irritability and stress levels;
- causes him to become intensely frustrated at being unable to correctly or perfectly execute something associated with his passion;
- causes him to lash out verbally or physically should you try to redirect him away from his activity;
- makes him withdraw from loved ones;
- makes him retreat more and more into activities affiliated with his passion;
- prevents him from completing necessary activities of daily life, such as dressing, bathing, or homework;
- takes precedence over being on time for school or other activities; or
- occupies his thoughts and dominates his conversation.

If you ascertain that your child's passion has gotten out of hand and is causing him harm, please consult with your pediatrician or request a referral to a qualified mental health professional. This does not mean you have to remove the passion entirely; it just means that, for whatever reason, it has become bigger than your child can manage and requires clinical support to balance it so that the passion can become pleasurable once more.

Should I allow my child to be involved in her passion as much as she wants?

None of us is able to be productive if we live life as a total hedonist, doing precisely what we wish to and nothing else all day every day—we would never work, take care of ourselves, or be available to our loved ones. We would also become disconnected from the real world, self-absorbed and isolated—this is a caution for any one of us, but especially for the child with autism who naturally chooses solitary activities.

Autism or no autism, your child is first and foremost a kid, *your child*; and you wouldn't permit any of your children to do whatever they want as often as they wish. As a parent, you have the right to expect your child with autism to fulfill obligations and responsibilities within the parameters you set forth as a parent. The issue here is one of *fair compromise*; not situation-by-situation bargaining, as some parents do, but visually setting limits via a chart or schedule that indicates to your child the times and opportunities she has on a daily basis to engage in her passion. On either side of these opportunities should be the obligations you expect her to fulfill, be it a household chore or school-related work. When you and your child agree to such an arrangement, you are in a better position to exert your parental authority when firmness is required. More on this is in the Fair Discipline chapter (Chapter 9).

My son's passion is the computer and video games—should I limit him to two hours a day?

If you are wondering whether you should impose a time constraint on your son's computer activities, chances are you're doing so because it has already become an issue of concern. Computer video games can have an addictive quality to them; to the child with autism in perfectionism mode, they may be perceived as a challenging affront that must be conquered at all costs, making it difficult or impossible to pull him away without a strong reaction like a blowout or meltdown. It is unclear if it is even possible to totally master any given video game, so your child's frustration level may be exacerbated by his perception of failure as the difficulty of the game increases.

Only you are in a position to determine if your son's computer video game interest is a healthy passion or an unhealthy obsession. If you believe it is a passion that simply requires your parental interference to safely retrieve your son, discuss your concerns with him (not while he's on the computer) and talk about the concept of fair compromise tempered with the obligations you expect of him. It may mean that you collaborate in building computer time into a visual schedule so that it is clear what needs to come before and after. You can aid your child in feeling like a partner in the process by allowing him to set a timer when he is on the computer so that he can visually track how much time he's got left before the time you both agreed on runs out. Follow your intuition and use your best parental judgment on how much time is too much; if all else fails, remember that as a parent you have the right to block or ban anything from your home that you feel is unhealthy for your child or your family.

How come my child doesn't want to share his passion with me, only with strangers?

If your child gravitates to strangers to share his passion, it likely results from ways in which you have historically responded to his desire to engage you. If you have perceived his passion as an obsession, a nuisance, or a clinical trait of autism that should be ignored in order to be treated, you have taught your child that what he so cherishes is unworthy of your time and consideration.

What your child probably gets from strangers (who don't regularly hear about the passion 24/7) is curiosity, indulgence, and, perhaps, genuine interest; in some instances, your child's interactions with adults about his passion may be a mutually shared interest! This, of course, can be corrected by your willingness to listen and participate the next time you observe your child enjoying his passion. One mom realized she had been communicating rejection every time her son approached her to share his interest in snakes, a subject she found unappealing. In desiring to reconnect with him, this mom is now as much of an expert—well, almost—as her son!

Should I use my child's passion as a reward to be earned?

Making your child earn her passion is a subjective judgment call that may set up a disaster situation for both you and your child. While you may believe you are creating an incentive for your child, you may really be effecting a lose–lose situation based on your expectations of what you think your child should accomplish.

Remember the "Simon Says" exercise discussed in Chapter 4 in which you were asked to participate? What if the one thing you truly loved in life was dependent on your ability to execute those instructions precisely in order to earn it? Obviously you failed to achieve the outcome expected of you because your senses were being assaulted concurrent with the instruction. Now, what if your passion is not for a thing but for a person—your very child. Because you didn't perform as expected, you didn't earn your passion for the day, and you forfeit time with your child. Reverse this in your child's instance, and you have a situation that will not only make your child feel frustrated and hopeless but embittered.

There may be a variety of reasons why your child is unable to attain the expectations set for her, but, as you have been learning, how much of it comes down to understanding her way of being and making compassionate accommodations versus her demonstration of willful misconduct?

Should I punish my child by withholding his passion?

It may be very tempting to withhold your child's passion as a punishment, especially if it seems as though nothing else has anywhere near as much impact—but kindly refrain from doing so, and here's why. There is precious little in your child's life over which he has any control. As someone with autism who is struggling to exist in an intolerant, overwhelming world, your child's passion is the one constant—one of the few things that he can not only control, but finds entirely and absorbingly satisfying as an intellectual and creatively stimulating outlet.

By removing your child's ability to access his passion, you are teaching disempowerment by demonstrating that, ultimately, you are in control of it, not your child. The uncertainty of when, where, and how the passion will be removed may create anxiety in your child or an unwillingness to reveal elements of his passion. It may also sow the seeds that could breed contempt and distrust.

In the spirit of fair compromise, it is acceptable to exert your parental authority by withholding special privileges pertaining to the passion, like disallowing a TV program or an extracurricular activity or event—but never suppress the passion itself in its entirety, nor your child's ability to access it of his own free will.

What do I do if, in the past, I have punished my child by terminating her passion?

It is not too late to go back and make it right in the same way that you would express remorse for having offended anyone in your life. Approach your child privately, gently, and respectfully and admit that you have been wrong and that you are learning. Confess that you have, in the past, assumed control over your child's most passionate of interests by taking it away; and pledge to reinstate it in full, to participate in it with your child, and not to consider suppressing it in its entirety again. If you make this commitment genuinely and sincerely, you should see a mending of trust amid the mutually pleasing opportunities that present themselves to you both in the future.

Is it okay for my child to have lots of "online friends" and play lots of online games?

The Internet has been a tremendous gift to people with autism who have difficulty with social interactions and communicating effectively in person. Connecting with others by using the computer levels the social playing field; everyone is equalized, or at least gets a fair chance without regard to social awkwardness or faux pas. Connecting with others who share their passion via computer is a social outlet your child may not otherwise experience anywhere else, one that can lead to long-lasting relationships.

Having said that, here is the concern expressed by one parent about her son's online acquaintances: "This seems to be a great way for him to communicate with others and is his preferred method. I am torn about allowing him as much time as he wants on the computer and forcing him to communicate with the rest of the family when he so obviously prefers the computer."

The intervention here is twofold. First, it is absolutely necessary to monitor very carefully with whom your child is interacting, with the same cautions of which we all must be aware when using the Internet. It is particularly important for this situation because, as someone who is likely very honest and direct, your child may be oblivious to someone's ulterior motives and divulge personal and private information. Discuss this in detail and visually post on the computer a checklist of topics or items that your child is forbidden to answer, or discuss together what appropriate comeback phrases might be. Second, as a parent you have the right to regulate the amount of time your child spends on the computer, as was previously discussed. To ensure fairness, arrange these conditions with your child well in advance, and agree to the expectations you have both put forth collaboratively.

How do I respond when my child's teacher says his need to talk about his passion is disruptive?

Your child's need to talk about his passion to the point of disruption is likely not an issue about the passion as much as it is a social issue. If your child flounders socially and has difficulty making those kinds of connections, it may be that discussing his passion is the one way he believes he can initiate conversation with his peers (and educators), thinking all the while that everyone shares his level of interest.

Find out exactly what your child's teacher means when he or she uses the term *disruptive*. Does it mean that the education of other children is being infringed? Or is it that the teacher finds your child's daily diatribes to be a personal annoyance? If the former, then it really is an issue to discuss with your child by setting visual limits, by showing him in person and through words and pictures, in terms of when and where he may discuss his passion (recess, lunchroom, free time). His teacher can help to reinforce these concepts as well. But if you feel your child's teacher simply does not understand your child's attempts to socially connect with others, try brainstorming ways to be proactive in supporting those connections during the agreed-on times when your child may engage in his passion during the day. Your child's teacher is in the very best position to know if there is any other child—even just one—who shares your child's passion.

How do I handle it when my child's passion seems to be isolating him socially because it is no longer appropriate for his age?

If your child's passion for something others may label "age inappropriate" remains steady and constant in spite of his age and the ever-changing interests of his peers, you may wish to intervene gently and sensitively. Let's face it—at a certain age, your child's interest in cartoons, *Barney*, or Yu-Gi-Oh is most likely going to stigmatize him. Let's be clear: this is not about extinguishing your child's passion, it's about tailoring and fine-tuning where, when, and with whom it is discussed until such time as the world is less judgmental.

Consider the following strategies:

- Your child can only know what he knows. In what ways have you exposed him to other opportunities, other experiences, in order to develop new passions that might better suit his age level?
- Have you carefully dissected the passion, or does it symbolize something greater that can be expressed in other ways?
- Is it possible to take related elements of your child's passion and translate them into a new passion that others may find more acceptable?
- Have you been able to facilitate helping your child connect with

at least one other person who shares his passion (in person or online)? It may be that you agree to reserve "passion chat" to times your child is able to share it with this person.

- Is there a way your child can spin an air of sophistication where his passion is concerned by discussing it from the standpoint of an historian, collector, or researcher?

Additionally, you may need to partner with your child to set boundaries about at-school versus at-home and after-school activities with people who love and understand him best.

Can my child's passion be used as a learning tool?

One way to validate your child's passion and approach it proactively is to understand its potential use to demystify education curriculum your child finds challenging. This tactic may also aid in shifting the way in which a resistant teacher perceives the passion. It is not realistic to expect that any educator teach to one student, but you, a classroom aide, or a learning support professional can help your child to deconstruct that which she is struggling to learn using her passion. There can be several benefits to doing this:

- You are breaking down something frustrating and reframing it in familiar terms.
- You are making learning fun and enjoyable.
- Your child is instantly engaged and ready to learn.
- Your child experiences academic success.
- Your relationship with your child, and your child's professional working relationships, are strengthened.

For example, maybe a child who loved the game *Mario Brothers* was having difficulty learning about plant life until it was explained that he would be appreciating plants similar to the hanging vines in his video game. Another child loved oceanography but struggled with mathematic concepts until he was told to picture dolphins as the numeric equivalents of the numbers in his math problems. Determining creative solutions such as these does not rest squarely on your shoulders alone; partner with your child and her professional team members to brainstorm unlimited possibilities.

Is it possible for my child's passion to become her job one day?

It is a distinct possibility that your child's passion could translate into employment—in fact, the future of her livelihood as an adult depends on your ability to nurture and cultivate her special interests and value them as worthwhile. The most famous example of a person with autism becoming not only viably employed but famously so is Temple Grandin.

Grandin's early intrigue with animals coupled with her creation of a gentle-pressure "squeeze machine" led her to develop improvements in the cattle industry by redesigning ways to calm and contain cattle in holding areas—in the same way she quelled her own anxieties. Her ability to rightfully speculate animals' needs, paired with her visualization capabilities, has led to her demand as an international presenter and respected author.

Identify your child's passions early on, and be prepared to follow wherever they might lead.

Will my child's passion hinder him from developing romantic relationships some day?

Your child's passion may actually be the catalyst that develops a relationship into a romance. Remember the importance of trying to connect your child with someone who shares his passion? Well, romance requires just one other person; and one person is all it takes to found a loving, pleasing, mutually satisfying relationship that may progress into longevity.

You've heard people's strong areas of special interest referred to as a "labor of love." Love is the tie that binds, and a mutual love can conjoin two people in the context of a shared passion. This makes sense when we consider the ways in which *anyone* typically develops a romance; it's usually through vocational, avocational, educational, or relationship contacts. There's no reason why the same couldn't hold true for your child with autism, and his passion makes a logical starting point.

How do I help others to see the value of my child's passion when they often see it as a nuisance or OCD?

Discuss your child's passion within the context of the presumption of intellect. Talk about all the good things that have come of your child's area of special interest, and how much you've benefited by learning about a subject for which you had no previous working knowledge. Share examples of your child's inspired creations stemming from his most passionate interest, and elaborate on the sense of elation and accomplishment your child radiates when engaged in fabricating his drawings, models, computer animations, or whatever it is that he so dearly loves. Finally, be certain to highlight any social encounters that have been facilitated as a result of your child's passion. Don't press an aggressive agenda, but do be respectfully persistent. Do not surrender to the notion that your child's passion is without value.

Is my child gifted in his passion?

We are all blessed with great gifts and natural talents—all of us. It may appear as though your child is "gifted" in his area of special interest; it's more likely that he is simply deeply vested in absorbing all he can about it, and this is how he prefers to spend his time. This doesn't make him a savant for his passion; just someone whose intellect is intact, and who is driven by a desire to learn and create at a young age. If a descriptor is to be used, perhaps the word *prodigy* is less sensational.

Because your child has the diagnosis of autism, which is considered debilitating by some, there's a certain awe factor inherent in the child who, outwardly, appears to be severely impaired and yet demonstrates an unusually skilled aptitude in one or more areas. Those misguided individuals who rush to label your child as "gifted" require a lecture about the presumption of intellect, and the theory that we are all more alike than different (although the awe factor is pretty cool while it lasts).

What can I do to further encourage my child's passion?

Within fair compromise and parental expectations, do all that you can to nurture and cultivate your child's passion as long as it continues to be an area of special interest and brings her great pleasure. And start young. Do not hesitate to pursue pilgrimages to museums, displays, and exhibitions; consult with professionals in that field (including university staff); or enroll your child in classes either in person or online. Look for opportunities to illuminate the fruit of your child's creativity through websites, message boards, and listservs, or by contributing to newsletters and publications specific to your child's area of special interest.

The child who thinks in pictures will carefully store and replay the memories from these moments for future use. Do not underestimate the influence these activities have in not only developing your child's talent, but in strengthening her confidence and self-esteem.

Chapter 8

TREATMENT OPTIONS

- Are treatments available to cure my child's autism or make it go away?
- My child's doctor recommends behavior therapy for my child—what is that?
- How long will my child need to be in therapy?
- I'm told my child needs FBA—what does that mean?
- I'm addressing my child's special dietary needs as well as her communication needs—isn't this all the therapy she needs?
- What is ABA?
- What is Lovaas?
- What is TEACCH?
- What is rapid prompting?
- What is Greenspan or floortime?
- What is RDI?
- What is social skills training?
- What are social stories?
- Why might a child who appears to have more challenges when very young end up having fewer of them when he is older?
- Why do some children respond to treatments and others don't?
- What causes some children to regress in their skills?
- How do I know what type of therapy is right for my child?
- What do I do if my child screams and tantrums before, during, and after therapy?
- Who pays for treatment therapies?
- I'm a single working mom and feel pressured and stressed to do all the new things I'm being asked to do—help!
- I feel like I need to bombard my child with as much therapy as possible in order for her to make gains—is this right?
- Am I wrong to look forward to my child's therapy time as a break to get household chores done?
- My child's therapist uses all kids of devices and toys I can't afford—what should I do?
- How do I handle it when my child's therapist visits and my other children seem to want her attention too?
- What can I do if I need help on the weekends and my child's therapist only works weekdays?
- Are there alternatives to the more traditional therapies?

Are treatments available to cure my child's autism or make it go away?

Most often when we hear of parents who claim their child has been "cured" of autism, what they really mean is that their child has received some sort of treatment that has enabled the child to decrease, modulate, regulate, or suppress his autism-instinctive responses to environmental stimuli and social interactions, which may include communications that get labeled as noncompliant or behavioral outbursts. Outwardly such kids appear to function "normally" and with the adherence to social norms that parents and educators would expect of most other children. This does not mean, however, that they are without autism or autistic features. Accomplishing this degree of compliance may be possible for some children with autism; it is an unlikely prospect for all, and depends on the will of the child to cooperate, and how stringently his parents maintain such standards of compliance.

Children with autism certainly require the familiar safety of structure and predictable routine; but as more autism self-advocates emerge from the adult world, we are hearing their perspective about "cure" and "recovery" from autism. They have been vocal in clearly communicating themes of acceptance, compassion, and sensitivity; however, few to none are actively advocating any method of treatment that promotes a "cure." Controversy over the ways to "recover" from autism may still prevail for some time to come, but it is generally acknowledged that autism is a lifelong experience, a natural way of being, and one of a myriad of variations on being human.

My child's doctor recommends behavior therapy for my child—what is that?

Behavior therapy is the practice of modifying, reducing, or eliminating "undesirable" or maladaptive behavior while reinforcing behavior that is deemed "acceptable." In the history of treating persons with developmental disabilities, who have so often been misunderstood, behavior therapy has translated into behavior management and control involving methods to chemically sedate and physically restrain individuals into submission. Such tactics of enforcing compliance have largely been discouraged in recent times, but still often occur in some clinical and educational settings.

When your child's doctor recommends behavior therapy, find out more about what he means. Is he referring to a specific type of treatment (read on for details) or is he speaking in generalized terms? Is the focus on ceasing your child's extreme behaviors as opposed to understanding your child's behaviors as communications? Remember that when your child acts out, it may be attributed to raging frustration at being unable to communicate in ways that are effective, reliable, and universally understandable. This extends to being unable to communicate physical pain and discomfort (including sensory sensitivities), as well as mental health issues separate from your child's autism (including acute anxiety). Merely seeking to extinguish behavior without understanding its cause does not presume your child's intellect and, in essence, does not address the real issues, but instead conceals them.

How long will my child need to be in therapy?

Should you decide to enroll your child in therapy, she will need to be in therapy until she demonstrates her ability to apply the therapy principles she's been learning on her own and across all aspects of her typical daily routines, without the verbal or physical prompting of a paid professional. When your child progresses to this point, the therapist should recognize her achievement and either discharge her from service or collaborate with you to craft a new plan of support that builds on your child's newly acquired strengths. This may involve transitioning to another therapist or professional who may hold expertise in a certain discipline.

From the outset, the therapist should set long- and short-term goals for your child that fit within a time frame leading to the conclusion of service. The goals should correlate with bringing your child up to par with the cognitive and developmental skill levels of her peers. In other words, be mindful of any plan of treatment that is open ended and without goals and timelines for achieving new skills.

If your child is consistently unable to meet therapy goals, you may wish to reevaluate exactly what is expected of your child and how the therapy is being delivered. For instance, is it taking into account how she best communicates, thinks, learns, and processes information and sensory stimuli? You may also wish to explore working with another therapist if you feel dissatisfied. Your child's therapy should not last indefinitely, and should be readily replicated by you and other members of your family.

I'm told my child needs FBA—what does that mean?

FBA refers to *functional behavior analysis* or *functional behavior assessment*, a process by which your child is observed by a behavior specialist (someone with background and experience in understanding child psychology and possibly the unique needs of kids with autism) in order to determine the function or source of your child's "behavior," so that a treatment plan of intervention can be devised. (You should also be interviewed during the FBA.) This process is usually recommended for children with behaviors that are challenging to understand and support (though always keep in mind that they may be just a form of communication). In some instances, the federal Individuals with Disabilities Education Act (IDEA) requires school districts to conduct an FBA on such children.

To be effective, your child should be observed in his natural environment (the place where he would ordinarily spend time), whether that is home or school, so that the behavior specialist may gather accurate information based on the ABCs of antecedent, behavior, and consequence. The *antecedent* pertains to the event(s) immediately preceding what results in the "behavior." The *behavior* is the manner in which your child reacts to the antecedent, and the *consequence* is whatever would typically occur as a result of the behavior exhibited. Here is an example: Your child indicates he wants cookies right before supper and you say no (antecedent), which causes your child to scream (behavior), which leads to you either caving in or standing your ground by applying some measure of discipline (consequence).

As you can see from the example, the ABCs can apply to *any* child, his learned behavior, and a parenting reaction that either reinforces undesirable behavior or teaches through discipline. To develop the most effective plan of support, the person conducting the FBA should temper a behavioral-based approach with a sensitive understanding of autistic "behavior" as an expression of communication so that the focus is on modifying your child's reactions, not terminating them without an understanding of their function.

I'm addressing my child's special dietary needs as well as her communication needs—isn't this all the therapy she needs?

There have been instances in which parents of children with autism have been pleasantly surprised by the improvements their children have made as a result of implementing a special dietary program for their child (refer to Chapter 5, Physical Well-Being). The advances reported have included greater ability to focus and concentrate, enhanced mood, and refinements in communication such as improved verbal speech or the initiation of speech.

Speech therapy may also be of great benefit for the child not yet articulating or the child who is challenged in speaking clearly and reliably. People with autism who were previously unable to communicate prior to speaking, or who discovered a viable speech alternative, often use the word *hell* to describe their frustration for the time they were mute.

Both approaches may yield significant advantages for your child, or they may have little to no effect. Although proper and thorough assessment of your child's needs (consultation with a nutritionist and speech therapist in this example) should guide you in making anticipatory decisions, there is no guarantee that any approach taken will be all your child requires in the way of support.

What is ABA?

Applied behavior analysis (ABA) is an intervention model that uses behavioral treatment approaches to provide intensive therapy in the form of specific training techniques. The therapy uses the FBA antecedent–behavior–consequence approach to creating opportunities for children with autism to learn and acquire skills (behavioral or academic) while discouraging and minimizing undesired behavior through the use of reinforcers. Reinforcers, which reward a proper response, may be verbal ("Good job!") or tangible (a toy or favored food item). For example, to learn the word *dog*, a therapist might hold a photograph or figurine of a dog and ask the child to correctly identify the subject while keeping the child attentive to the task (instead of engaging in distractions), and responding with praise for proper response and good attending behavior. Criteria for success and achievement of goals is measured in terms of desired versus nondesired responses given by the child. ABA is delivered to a child one on one by a trained therapist or a paraprofessional (someone supervised by an accredited professional) in intensive segments of time ranging anywhere from twenty-five to forty or more hours a week.

In the best circumstances, the principles learned by a child in ABA should be adapted to environmental situations beyond the isolated encounters with a professional. Acknowledgment should also be given to opportunities for the child with autism to play and learn in his natural environment, and to be afforded time to just be a kid by interacting with siblings and peers. ABA therapy is considered most efficacious for children between the ages of two and six years old, and may last up to two years.

ABA is considered a scientific method of intervention because studies have been conducted that validate its procedures of improved behavior in children with autism through the research of practitioners. You may also hear ABA referred to as *behavior therapy*, *intensive behavioral treatment*, *discrete trial training*, and *Lovaas*. The Association for Behavior Analysis website address is www.abainternational.org.

What is Lovaas?

Lovaas is named after O. Ivaar Lovaas (pronounced E-var Low-vahhs), the University of California at Los Angeles Psychology Department professor who began working with children with autism in the early 1960s and, in the 1980s, made publicly available his approaches to aid children with autism to regain speech, advance educationally, and adopt proper behavioral conduct. In so doing, Lovaas established an intensive method of treating autistic symptoms through discrete trial training or a repetition of tasks and lessons that reinforce positive responses and negate noncompliant ones. This technique is considered ABA, yet differs in that it not only requires intensive one-on-one interaction with the child with autism for a minimum of forty hours weekly, but parents are expected to participate so that twenty-four-hour consistency is provided.

There are a few things to consider, however, before implementing the Lovaas method:

- Dr. Lovaas has published studies in scientific peer-reviewed journals in which he suggests that young children with autism that participated in his program are "recoverable" or curable, which is a matter of debate
- The professional delivering the intervention must have received training from the Lovaas Institute in one of its West or East Coast offices, because only this person is qualified to implement the program.
- Because of the highly trained and qualified personnel, the program is costly to implement as recommended.
- In its earliest incarnation, a child's negative responses were responded to forcefully with angry words, a slap, or a swat on the head; this aversive approach is no longer supposed to be a component of treatment.

However, due to the thoroughness of his data collection and the purported improvements in some children with autism he's treated, Dr. Lovaas has a great following of many supporters including parents, professionals, and academicians. In 1981, he published *The ME Book: Teaching Developmentally Disabled Children* as a manual to aid parents and professionals training children with autism in verbal imitation, self-care skills, and advanced language. Catherine Maurice's book, *Let Me Hear Your Voice: A Family's Triumph over Autism*, documents her positive experiences in treating her two children with the Lovaas method. For further information about Dr. Lovaas and his method, check out www.lovaas.com

What is TEACCH?

TEACCH is the acronym for Treatment and Education of Autistic and Related Communication of Handicapped Children, an autism program that is a division of the University of North Carolina (UNC) at Chapel Hill Department of Psychiatry. TEACCH was initiated in the early 1970s by founder Dr. Eric Schopler, professor of psychiatry and psychology at UNC for more than forty years, and a pioneer in the delivery of respectful and humane treatment of individuals with autism.

TEACCH focuses its approach on the child with autism as an individual with unique interests, skills, and needs, and tailors a person-centered program that builds on those existing strengths in order to cultivate, adapt, and accommodate the acquisition of new skills. TEACCH emphasizes as its philosophy that individuals with autism have a unique culture that, although different, is similar to—but not inferior to—that of the rest of us.

Training in the TEACCH modality and approach occurs at regional centers located in North Carolina; most of the referrals to TEACCH come from within the state, with up to 10 percent from out of state or from other countries. TEACCH claims that it prepares young children with autism for inclusion in typical school settings and integration into community life for adults at a rate of 5 percent need for "institutionalization," as compared to the international average of 46 percent. For further information about TEACCH, visit the website at www.teacch.com.

What is rapid prompting?

Rapid prompting is a method predicated on the belief that individuals with autism who also have apraxia (the inability to reliably articulate and properly sequence spoken language) are able to communicate fluently if taught to point to letters or a keyboard arranged in alphabetical order. In time, skills for writing and typing are introduced with the intended goal being one of independent response. Rapid prompting differs from facilitated communication (see the communication chapter, Chapter 3) in that there is no physical touch, or facilitation, involved.

Rapid prompting was developed by Soma Mukhopadhyay, mother to son Tito, who refused to believe that her son was without an intact intellect despite being told by doctors in their native country, India, that Tito would never learn. Soma abandoned a career in chemistry in order to work intensively with Tito by building on his passion (in Tito's example, an interest in numbers on a calendar), constant narration of their mutual activities, educating him at or beyond his age level, and rubber-banding a pencil to his fingers in order draw and write. In rapid prompting, an individual's extraneous movements or visual distractions are disregarded in favor of keeping them focused on the activity at hand using the combination of preceding techniques to elicit proper responses that reveal the child's true intellect through a barrage of stimulating input.

Training for the rapid prompting method takes place at the HALO (Helping Autism through Learning and Outreach) clinic in Austin, Texas. For further insight into rapid prompting, read Tito's book, *The Mind Tree: A Miraculous Child Breaks the Silence of Autism*, and check out www.halo-soma.org.

What is Greenspan or floortime?

The Greenspan or floortime treatment approach was devised by Dr. Stanley Greenspan, a child psychiatrist and professor of psychiatry, behavioral sciences, and pediatrics at George Washington University Medical School. (Dr. Greenspan is also the founder of the Zero to Three: National Center for Infants, Toddlers and Families.) Dr. Greenspan has collaborated with Serena Weider, a clinical psychologist, to expand the array of services building from Dr. Greenspan's philosophies.

Floortime is an intensive one-on-one intervention that seeks to engage children with autism by building on the relationship established when parents get down on the floor (hence the name) to interact with their children during playtime. The emotional reactions elicited between parent and child lead to learning opportunities within the context of the relationship (for example, pointing to a toy and encouraging the child to communicate her desire for it). It is considered a spontaneous and joyful "practice time" that naturally motivates a child to learn through her interests.

Two adjunct components of this process are working with various therapists from a range of disciplines who use the floortime model to foster further development within the context of therapeutic strategies, and working with parents to adjust or refine their approach to interacting with their child. For further information on floortime, go to www.floortime.org; for details about Dr. Greenspan, visit www.stanleygreenspan.com.

What is RDI?

RDI stands for *relationship development intervention*, a method that, according to its founder, psychologist Dr. Steve Gutstein, provides the majority of people on the autism spectrum with the ability to achieve a "true quality of life." Dr. Gutstein created RDI in reaction to the challenges he faced in authentically replicating traditional one-on-one autism treatments across environments; he discovered his clients' inability to translate much of what they had learned outside of therapy to typical environments.

RDI has as its guiding principles a focus on quality of life within the context of caring relationships and dynamic environments. This is achieved through mastering everyday activities, using a variety of communication options, developing pleasing memories linked to learning opportunities, and continually challenging children with autism to expand their experiences by tapping what Dr. Gutstein calls their *dynamic intelligence.*

RDI targets core deficits in individual children in order to remediate those attributes by nurturing strengths and relationships. Parents are encouraged to attend a Houston, Texas–based four-day orientation seminar, after which they are referred to an RDI specialist for continuing follow-up. Ongoing video evaluation and other support are offered. For learn more about RDI, check out www.rdiconnect.com.

What is social skills training?

Social skills training operates from the premise that an autistic lack of social and emotional reciprocity is more about a lack of know-how than it is about social disinterest. The theory is that an individual with autism generally avoids social situations due to performance anxiety or stigmatizes himself through well-intentioned but inappropriate social faux pas. Social skills training seeks to break down and instruct such individuals in the "art of people," much like an anthropologist studying a culture. This may occur through:

- identifying areas of social challenge;
- observation of typical social interactions (videotaped, staged, or in real time);
- creative problem solving;
- modeling acceptable behavior;
- teaching tips, hints, and strategies;
- learning about feelings and emotions;
- understanding social idioms such as slang and sarcasm;
- decoding body language;

- practicing appropriate interactions through role-playing/role-reversal;
- developing scripts to initiate, sustain, or close social conversation;
- videotaping and deconstructing areas of need and successes; and
- revisiting, tweaking, and fine-tuning social strategies.

Social skills training can occur one on one, in a group of peers, or with a mentor (an adult who facilitated learning). To learn more, you may wish to begin by checking out www.modelmekids.com, or read Kathleen Quill's book *Do-Watch-Listen-Say*.

What are social stories?

Social stories are written and/or pictorially scripted scenarios to support the child with autism who best retains information via visual means in a concrete, sequential, and repetitive format. Such narratives may explain social protocols (such as handshaking or eye contact), demystify circumstances that may create fear or anxiety, deconstruct the rationale or sequence of various processes, aid in preparing someone for knowing what's coming next, and support an understanding of what to expect and what is expected in social settings. It is important that a social story reinforce the good things a child does currently and seek to improve on that; it is a misuse of a social story is to punish, manage, or control a child's behavior for the sake of compliance.

The concept of social stories was developed in 1991 by Carol Gray, a Michigan special educator and consultant to students with autism. Examples of social stories promoted by Gray as effective include self-care skills, time concepts (waiting, hurrying), community-based events (various appointments and chores), weather systems, holidays, and socially acceptable behavior. Gray also created *comic strip conversations*, another way of teaching social understanding in comic-panel format using voice balloons and thought bubbles to help define what others are saying and possibly thinking in social encounters.

To find out more about social stories and comic strip conversations, visit The Gray Center for Social Learning and Understanding at www.thegraycenter.org.

Why might a child who appears to have more challenges when very young end up having fewer of them when he is older?

That a child shows fewer challenges as he grows and matures could be attributable to one or a combination of several factors:

- proper diagnosis or reassessment of diagnosis,
- improved quality of family relationships,
- connecting with a loving and patient mentor,
- finding the proper method(s) of treatment and support,
- building on personal passions,
- development of communication and self-expression skills,
- fostering enhanced social connections,
- identification of the source for physical pain and discomfort, and
- identification and proper treatment of adjunct mental health issues.

In addition, despite all the brilliance and expertise of parents and professionals who desire to be of service, there are those children with autism who figure out—on their own—how to blend and assimilate in order to get by and fit in. This occurs through very careful observation of the behavior of others in person, on television, and in movies and cartoons. This kind of drive to participate is a tremendous strength, and should be recognized, acknowledged, and validated as such—it is hard work trying to replicate a reasonable facsimile of socially acceptable behavior. It is also a noble endeavor on the part of those children who independently come to the grave realization that the world best accommodates those who are perceived as "normal."

Why do some children respond to treatments and other don't?

Children with autism will respond differently to different methods, approaches, techniques, and treatments because one size does not fit all. That is, there is no one single mode of treatment that can claim it has been proven effective in successful remediation of *all* children with autism. Remember that autism is a unique and individual experience, just as each individual is unique.

If what works for one child does not work for another, it will require that an alternative course of action be revised and developed to best accommodate that child's distinct way of being, way of learning, and way of processing the world. This can lead to a frustrating course of trial and error in seeking a solution; but it is necessary in order to willingly engage the child in a treatment program suited to meet her individual requirements.

It is not advisable to simply persist in enforcing a treatment program that has not been effective; this may only drive the child further from it, or will teach the child compliance without a working knowledge base. Any sound method of treatment should have, as a key component, the aptitude for adaptation and flexibility.

What causes some children to regress in their skills?

Some children with autism may appear to regress or lose previously acquired skills for a variety of reasons. Could it be that their autism is compromised still further by another neurological issue that has gone undetected? Is it because no one has presumed the intellect of the child, and so he is, in essence, giving up by reflecting back what others project on him? Or has he developed a "learned helplessness" that can develop when someone does everything for him, as one would care for an infant—without presuming intellect or teaching the acquisition of new skills?

Additional reasons why some children may regress in their skills could include:

- growing frustration with the inability to communicate;
- emotional anxiety or distress due to home, school, or community issues;
- overwhelming physical pain and discomfort;
- undiagnosed mental health issues, including depression and post-traumatic stress;
- poor working relationship with therapists, educators, and other professionals;
- misunderstanding and misinterpretation of what is expected;
- a vacation from school or therapy during which newly acquired skills were not made functional and were permitted to languish; and
- continuing treatment that's not a good fit with the child.

If your child has regressed or lost previously acquired skills, do not hesitate to arrange an immediate appointment with your child's pediatrician for evaluation and assessment of any of the above areas of concern, in addition to any areas of concern your doctor may have.

How do I know what type of therapy is right for my child?

Finding the right therapy or combination of therapeutic approaches is a process. Parents of newly diagnosed children often wish to take advantage of the plasticity of their young child's developing brain during the early years of their life (termed the "window of opportunity" by some). You may wish to consider the following questions when matching a treatment modality with the needs of your child:

- Is your child being harmed in any way, or is she engaged and involved?
- Is your life and that of your family more or less stressful as a result?
- Is the effectiveness of the therapy backed with scientific validation or research-based studies in published literature?
- Are there specific assessment procedures or ways to measure progress?
- Are there short- and long-term goals?
- Does the therapy incorporate your child's current strengths, skills, and passions?
- Can you or your family members readily replicate the therapy?
- Can the therapy be integrated into your child's other treatment or educational programs?
- Is the therapy "transportable" no matter where you and your child may be (i.e., grandma's house, vacation, at the airport)?
- Does the therapy not only teach new skills, but lead to expanded possibilities of existing skills?

In lieu of the synopses of previously discussed treatments, some savvy parents are opting for the "stew approach," which involves taking the best components of various therapies and blending them into one overarching approach stylized to meet the unique personality, strengths, and needs of their child. To further explore this concept, you may wish to partner with your child, your spouse, your child's doctor, and other professionals who can share their insight and experience about taking this eclectic path of treatment.

What do I do if my child screams and tantrums before, during, and after therapy?

Foremost, your child's verbal refusal, physical resistance, or acting out before, during, and after therapy should be interpreted by you, the parent, as a direct and clear communication that something is wrong. If your child has a way to communicate effectively and reliably, interview her in order to discern more information about what is wrong. Unless and until you ascertain precisely what is causing this kind of reaction in your child, carefully consider the immediate discontinuation of whatever therapy is inciting this sort of visceral response—otherwise, it is not worth risking the perpetuation of potential trauma for your child.

Your child's responses may be due to the lack of a trusting, respectful relationship with the attending professional, or the possibility that your child is expected to participate in something that is causing a painful (emotionally or physically) reaction. If you have been participating in treatment sessions (as is recommended so you can replicate the therapy), you may already hold suspicions about what could be wrong. Do not be intimidated into silent submission by any therapist's credentials, background, experience, or training. You are your child's parent, and you know your child better than anyone!

Consider simultaneously investigating the situation in the following manner. If you have been inconsistent in participating, and haven't immediately ceased therapy, make time to carefully observe all or a portion of your child's next therapy session (insist on it)—rely on your parenting instincts to guide you in knowing what does and does not feel right. Double-check with anyone you know who has observed the therapist in action with your child or other clients.

Next, compare your child's reactions with that of other people with whom he interacts—how is it dissimilar and what makes it so? Finally, interview the therapist to learn his or her impression of your child's reactions to treatment. If that professional dismisses your concerns because you haven't been trained (and he or she knows better), tells you it is normal, or downplays the severity of what is happening (saying your child will get used to it), it is probably time to locate a new therapist who is more compassionate and collaborative.

Who pays for treatment therapies?

If your child qualifies for participation in your state's Early Intervention program, your child's needs will determine the services provided, which may include therapy at no cost to you. Follow up with your county's Human Services office (in the community pages of your local telephone directory) for further details.

Insurance law is regulated on a state-by-state basis, so whether your child's services for treatment therapies will be covered by your health insurance will vary depending on your location. It may be that your health insurance covers a percentage of a particular therapy when prescribed by your child's physician. Other insurance plans may cover all or some therapy based on your child's need, which may not necessarily include autism (for example, speech therapy to address a speech delay). Some states have insurance laws that exclude autism altogether.

Depending on your income level or your child's developmental level, you may also qualify for Medicaid-funded services, which may include coverage of treatment therapies. Some insurers will discontinue covering therapeutic services once a child reaches school age, based on the understanding that responsibility shifts to the education system. Regardless of your insurance coverage, you may well need to pay for some or all of your child's therapy treatment, especially if you decide to hire a private therapist to deliver services to your child. Check with your employer for information about insurance coverage and limitations ("caps"). If you are in advocate mode, and frustrated by navigating insurance, you may voice your concerns directly to your state's insurance commissioner and other elected legislators.

I'm a single working mom and feel pressured and stressed to do all the new things I'm being asked to do—help!

During the initial visitation to meet and greet your child, a good therapist will thoroughly interview you and your family in your home, and at your convenience, in order to determine your family's coping style, strengths, and resources. Therapy should occur wherever your child happens to be, and in young kids this means your home or preschool. In addition to the services they can offer, the therapist may suggest:

- opportunities for parent education,
- contact information for local autism organizations,
- additional parent-to-parent connections,
- referral to other professionals that may be helpful, and
- available respite services so you can have time apart from your child.

Therapy should not be about heaping more on your already overflowing plate, complicating your life with unrealistic expectations—especially for the single parent. Also, although you are asked to participate in the delivery of supports to your child to ensure consistency, this should not be developed and implemented without your involvement, recommendations, and consent.

Any treatment plan that is developed for your child should meet with your approval, include contributions from you and your family, flow within your natural daily routines, be easily replicated, and should create less—not more—stress in your life as your child gains new skills and develops positive ways of coping. If you are at all over-whelmed by what any professional expects of you, do not feel shy or embarrassed to be vocal in communicating that it is too much or not top priority in the grand scheme of life. Respectfully request that what is expected of you be better modified to adapt to your lifestyle. Don't be guilt-tripped into complying if you're frazzled; treatment needs to make sense for your child *and* you.

I feel like I need to bombard my child with as much therapy as possible in order for her to make gains—is this right?

While is it understandable that you may wish to take advantage of your young child's developmental years, there is nothing to suggest that your child will benefit from around-the-clock therapy in order to advance and improve. Children need time to be kids and to be able to play freely, either alone or with siblings and other children. Your endeavor to support your child to the fullest should not morph into an obsessive overkill that will threaten to evoke stress, tension, and burnout in both you and your child.

Find a way to determine a healthy and reasonable balance, and focus on the quality and not quantity of therapy. Remember: therapy should not mean that your child's life has to come to a crashing halt in order to implement it. Any therapeutic method should be readily replicable by you, and should be able to occur within the flow of your family's natural daily routines. If it feels good, is fun, and takes place within the context of loving, respectful relationships, your child will be best poised for success.

Am I wrong to look forward to my child's therapy time as a break to get household chores done?

Parents of children with autism can have especially busy and complex lives, and time management can be very challenging. However, please remember that any therapy is intended to be temporary. In fact, the sooner therapeutic techniques are transferred to you, the child's parent, the sooner everyone will need to depend less on therapy. Therefore, it is important that you participate during your child's therapy time—provided in your home or a clinical setting—by observing, interacting with the therapist, and working with your child to replicate the therapy in your home. (Depending on your insurance or Early Intervention plan, your presence may actually be a requirement.)

As tempting as it may be, it is inappropriate to look on your child's therapy sessions as "baby-sitting" or a way for you to get chores done. In some instances, parents have even run neighborhood errands while the therapist is alone with their child. If you are desperate for time away, do not feel guilty about wanting time to yourself: a day to shop, a weekend out of town, or a quiet restaurant dinner. Your local Human Services agency may be able to provide you with contacts for nearby respite, comparable to highly qualified child care provided in the home of someone trained to support kids with physical and developmental differences.

My child's therapist uses all kinds of devices and toys I can't afford—what should I do?

Your child (and even her siblings) may really look forward to the arrival of the visiting therapist who brings lots of fun and interesting toys and other devices designed to engage and motivate your child. There is something to be said for the attraction of unusual spinning, light-up, noise-making toys designed and marketed by companies that cater to kids with disabilities of all kinds. (You may be shocked at just how expensive some such deceptively simple-appearing toys can cost.) If your child's therapist has an arsenal of toys not found in your own home, therapy days may be eagerly awaited events in your household.

But on reconsideration of therapy as a temporary support, you may wish to rethink the value of engaging your child with expensive equipment and toys—at least in ways that exclusively rely on those devices. If your child's therapist hasn't already interviewed you and assessed what you have available in your own home, express your concern about the inability to compete with the therapist's special equipment. It makes more sense—especially where replicating therapy is concerned—to adapt your child's existing living environment to playtime and therapy activities using what is already available. An expensive physical therapy ball could just as easily be supplanted with sofa cushions, and have the same effect. A costly cause-and-effect water toy for occupational therapy could just as easily be constructed at the kitchen sink using your household utensils.

In concert with your child and her therapist, brainstorm substitutes and alternatives to therapy equipment, toys, and devices so that there may be consistency and continuity in supporting your child beyond therapy sessions.

How do I handle it when my child's therapist visits and my other children seem to want her attention too?

When your child's therapist comes to visit, it may be a special and exciting time for him and his brothers or sisters who are curious, desire to be involved, and wish to help out. A strong therapist will be nonplussed by such attention, and will be flexible enough to use it to her advantage by fostering relationship-based interactions between your child and his siblings. For example, in a one-on-one scenario, the speech therapist might read a book with your child, and then elicit his enunciation of a specific word or name. With siblings also participating in the same setting, the therapist may allow a brother or sister to read the book to your child instead, or the therapist might encourage the sibling to elicit the correct response from your child. Even if, in exuberance, a sibling blurts out the answer to a question intended to be articulated by your child with autism, there is still an opportunity for your child to mimic or imitate the vocalization made familiar by one of your other children.

Such a scenario can translate to any variety of therapy situations, and should be welcomed, not discouraged, by the consulting therapist.

What can I do if I need help on the weekends and my child's therapist only works weekdays?

The key word in this question is *help*. Who is the help for—you or your child? And what kind of help is it that requires a therapist on the weekend? If you feel your child has a legitimate need—and this is an issue separate from any dependency, or wouldn't be better addressed through a respite program—ask any of your child's therapists if they can be flexible in their hours. It may be that such an arrangement is needed because of your hours or if your child spends time away from home and may suddenly need the therapist there.

Remember that, according to your insurance policy or Early Intervention program plan, you may only be permitted a set number of therapy hours a week unless you are funding additional time privately, so you should be mindful of not exceeding the hours allotted. Some therapists may be open to accommodating your weekend requests; some will not because they don't work weekends, have their own life on the weekends, are still going to school, or are working another job.

It is important to know that while the professionals in your child's life may be an important resource, therapists have other clients and should not be considered on call. Please appreciate that there is no such thing as a "therapy emergency" that would necessitate your need for weekend help. Whatever your child's therapist has imparted to you should be easily replicated by you and your family outside of therapy appointments.

Are there alternatives to the more traditional therapies?

Because no one medical cure or single treatment modality has proven effective for all children with autism, alternative and unconventional treatments for children on the autism spectrum abound. Your desire to explore such treatments may be driven by:

- hope that something "new" will help,
- reports or firsthand accounts of improvements from other parents,
- skepticism of scientifically based treatments,
- lack of finding a good fit with other treatments, or
- desiring to pursue more holistic resources.

Therapies that may be considered alternative may include various diets, chelation therapy (removal of internal metals and toxins), vitamin supplements, natural energy drinks, massage and acupuncture, vision treatments, hormone injections, and opportunities to swim with dolphins or ride horseback.

In exploring alternative treatments, bear in mind the concepts of presumption of intellect, prevention instead of intervention, building on passions, and relationship-based opportunities; sometimes the simplest, most natural solutions are the best. The preceding qualifications would seem ideally suited to the match made between one young man on the autism spectrum and his connection with his pet. His mom relates, "I know there are a lot of options out there from horse therapy to brushing techniques to chelation therapy. We have not really tried anything other than to keep good communication with Logan. One of the best things we ever did for Logan was get him a dog. The dog often acts as a buffer for him. When he has the dog with him, he is less anxious around people. They attend obedience school together and it has been one of the best experiences for Logan outside the home."

Chapter 9

FAIR DISCIPLINE

■ I was told that because my child has autism, I shouldn't discipline him because he doesn't know any better. Is this right?

■ What do I do when some of my relatives think my child is a brat who needs a good spanking?

■ Am I a bad parent if I can't get my child to behave?

■ I don't really have a discipline style per se—why should I adopt one now?

■ How do I handle it if my spouse thinks my child is being just plain manipulative?

■ Isn't it true that a lot of what my child does is being interpreted out of context?

■ Should I push my child in order to prepare him for the real world?

■ Who else should be allowed to discipline my child?

■ What do I do if I disagree with the way my spouse or my in-laws discipline my child?

■ How do I communicate my expectations to my child with autism?

■ How do I determine consequences for my child's behavior?

■ What is an appropriate way to discipline my child with autism?

■ Is spanking an appropriate way to discipline my child with autism?

■ How do I deal with my other kids thinking my child with autism is being given special treatment?

■ My child with autism talks and tries giving me lengthy explanations when I'm disciplining her—how do I deal with this?

■ Should I discipline my speaking child if I ask him to give me an explanation for something that happened and he won't say anything?

■ What can I do if my child's sense of justice and injustice seems very black and white and rigid?

■ How do I deal with it if my child tries applying his discipline rules to me and his siblings?

■ Am I wrong to tolerate my child pulling my hair or scratching me when I'm attempting to discipline her?

■ Do I discipline if my child melts down when one of my other children plays loud music, but he goes into his bedroom and plays music just as loudly?

■ How do I handle it when my child keeps running out of the house unattended?

■ Do I discipline my five-year-old child with autism any differently than my eleven-year-old with autism?

■ How do I handle it when I'm accused of being the only one who knows how to manage my child?

■ What do I do when I have been asked not to attend my place of religion due to my child's behavior?

■ What is the "dignity of risk"?

■ At what point will my child stop needing to be disciplined?

I was told that because my child has autism, I shouldn't discipline him because he doesn't know any better. Is this right?

All children need discipline, and your child with autism is no exception. Too often, the word *discipline* is associated with *punishment*, but the Latin root of the word *discipline* pertains to the act of teaching. Discipline should be approached from the perspective of teaching life lessons in order to prepare your child for what lies ahead.

Withholding discipline because you believe your child doesn't know any better does not presume your child's intellect, and the belief that he can learn—and it sets up a disservice to your child by being overprotective and creating artificial circumstances in which you bypass the opportunity to instruct your child in distinguishing right from wrong, as you would for any child. However, how you do this may look and sound differently than how you'd approach it for another child. Read on for further information.

What do I do when some of my relatives think my child is a brat who needs a good spanking?

The answer to this question really depends on how much time and effort you wish to invest in gently but persistently educating others about your child's way of being. How much do your relatives truly know about autism, or have they been unduly influenced by sensationalized media portrayals that present a biased or unfavorable perception? In approaching the situation from an educational standpoint, are there resources that you can provide your relatives that are simple, easy to understand, and explain autism in a way that will aid them in rethinking how they view your child? If you are pleased with this publication, or others, you may well wish to hand your relatives a copy (with a bookmark inserted in this chapter).

Remember that the genetic strand for autism spectrum traits may prevail on your family; this means you may have to rely on very clear-cut and visual information to convey essential tenets about autism to your relatives so as not to overwhelm them. The websites and recommended reading list at the back of this book might make a good start. Additionally, you may have seen a good video on autism or know of an upcoming conference or presentation that seems like it could broaden your relatives' understanding.

A number of popular television dramas and mainstream movies are featuring characters with autism in their plots—this might be an entrée into discussion as well (maybe starting with the example of *Rainman*). You may also wish to highlight myths and stereotypes about autism that were once believed as a way of broaching the "brat" dialogue, such as the theory that cold, indifferent "refrigerator" mothers induced their child's autism by withholding affection.

In what ways are you preparing your child for spending time with your relatives? Prevention instead of intervention can go a long way toward enhancing perceptions of any child who gets bored, agitated, or restless at family gatherings.

Finally, there are some people who you just may never be able to reach. Are you able to accept that as an option, even if it means being excluded from future get-togethers with your family?

Am I a bad parent if I can't get my child to behave?

This question requires deconstructing in two parts. First, the notion of being a bad parent—from where does this originate? Is it self-imposed because of struggles and frustrations over raising a unique child? Or is it coming from external sources (see the preceding question) that are making you feel as though you are failing to be an effective parent, or at least as effective as others expect of you? These are aspects to discern. If your feeling like a bad parent is self-imposed, it is likely that you would benefit from support in the form of compassionate counsel. This can be as informal as commiserating in person, by phone or online, with another parent of a child with autism who's "been there, done that" and who can relate to your attitude. Or it may be a more formal resource with which you might connect through your local Human Services agency, such as a family counselor, or a class to learn new parenting strategies.

The second part of the question pertains to being unable to get your child to behave. The respectful speculation here is that getting your child to "behave" refers to enforcing behavior compliance in the way that you might expect from other children who are acting out or behaving in ways that are very disruptive. As you've been reading the information in this book and other resources, you've surely been learning that we are all more alike than different, but that children with autism interpret and process information uniquely.

Reflect on those situations in which you have been unable to get your child to "behave," but now process what transpired by applying presumed intellect in addition to an understanding of your child's limitations of communication, possibly misperceived pain and discomfort (including sensory sensitivities), and undetected mental health issues, such as acute anxiety. Your child thrives on safety in sameness and predictable routine—was this present, suddenly removed, or altered without warning? Thoroughly applying the concept of prevention instead of intervention in concert with understanding in these areas may enable you to determine the source of your child's behavior. In deconstructing your child's most recent behavioral challenge, can you identify its source given what you've been learning using the "inside-out" perspective of this book as your resource?

I don't really have a discipline style per se—why should I adopt one now?

It is important to adopt a discipline style now because your child thinks and learns differently from most other children, so the techniques with which your parents disciplined you (like sending you to your room) are not likely to be effective or hold meaning for your child. The approach with which you were raised is probably also a subjective one, meaning that it is open to parental interpretation based on how most kids behave and personal experiences.

As you have been learning throughout this book, when you operate from the premise of presumed intellect, you'll better appreciate that your child has good reasons for doing what he's doing, and he's doing the best he knows how to in the moment. This position betters allows an objective or outside perspective in creatively interpreting the authentic rationale with which your child just demonstrated through actions, activities, and vocalizations that should foremost be interpreted as communications, not behaviors for bad behavior's sake. By presuming intellect, implementing a fair system of discipline, by being conscious and aware of your child's communication, and his pain and mental or emotional health needs, you and your child will both understand how to create the structure, routines and consistency required for successful good times.

How do I handle it if my spouse thinks my child is being just plain manipulative?

Kids are kids. And let's face it, manipulating one's parents to get what we want is a learned behavior that almost every child employs at some time in the history of their upbringing (some more than others). If this is true of your child, how did he learn it? From a sibling or from you? Any child will assume increasing amounts of control over his parents if he knows he can get away with it—the child with autism included.

If your spouse is right, the thing to determine is why your child is being manipulative; is it to get something he wants or is it to get a legitimate need met? For example, imagine being coerced into going to the store to get a toy you promised you'd buy, but having to interrupt the shopping trip to go home because of a tantrum due to his sensory sensitivities maxing out? In this example, the "want" was obtaining the toy, but the "need" was exiting from the environment.

The other aspect of this question to consider is that maybe your spouse disbelieves that your child is authentically autistic and that your child is merely playing you. Is it true that your child behaves better for your spouse because your spouse is a heavy-handed disciplinarian who brooks no nonsense? It's likely that any child would react to that sort of intimidation with compliance, but that doesn't resolve the issue of authentic autism—your child still experiences autism regardless of whether he complies better for your spouse than you! If your spouse is disbelieving of your child's autism, is it because your spouse is in denial or hasn't been as involved as you have been? Is it because your spouse's questions and concerns haven't been resolved? Has your spouse fully absorbed the impact of the autism diagnosis, or is your spouse perhaps blaming you for your child's way of being? These are issues to consider, together with revisiting the same strategies of outreach that you might use when educating relatives.

Isn't it true that a lot of what my child does is being interpreted out of context?

One good rule of thumb is to start addressing your child with autism's misbehavior by deconstructing it from the perspective that it is some form of communication. As you have been learning, even if your child with autism speaks, she may not have a way to describe or put language to what she is feeling. She may be unable to recognize her own escalating symptoms as they well up within her until it's too late, at which point she may deprecate herself with blame and frustration at being unable to hold it together.

Your child is never too young for you to begin instilling concepts of self-advocacy in your parenting style. Your child is a child first, but she is a child with a unique way of being that requires compassionate accommodations. Begin fostering self-advocacy early on and in ways your child will comprehend by making her aware of her autism, emphasizing the importance of communication (and communication alternatives), and helping her understand her sensitivities to sensory input, pain and discomfort, and anxiety-producing situations (and how to gain relief from such situations).

Lastly, your child will require you to advocate on her behalf until she is able to do so by aiding those around her to understand that her motives are often misinterpreted. This may be a very trying process—you must convince people to presume and respect your child's intellect instead of relying on old paradigms and stereotypes about "these kids."

Should I push my child in order to prepare him for the real world?

The answer to this question depends on how you define the phrase *push my child.* If you expect your child to comply through (conscious or unconscious) force or coercion because "it's for his own good," you are circumventing the principles put forth in this book, and you will best be served by finding some other resources on autism. What your child needs in order to prepare him for the world is sensitive understanding, compassionate accommodations, and patient opportunities to give back what he has to offer.

The world may, indeed, be harsh and cruel and oftentimes intolerant of people's differences. Your motives may well be intended in the spirit of giving your child every advantage; but in so pressuring your child, are you only adding to the very nature of the society that you seek to advantage your child against? Facing an insensitive world everyday is tough enough. More than anything, your child needs a safe and loving environment in which he is accepted and loved unconditionally and, within that forum, he can be taught how to equip himself in order to do his best to get by and fit in "out there."

Who else should be allowed to discipline my child?

Your child has the potential to be disciplined by anyone in whose company she finds herself when she is not in your direct presence. This may include:

- your spouse,
- your other children,
- your parents,
- your in-laws,
- extended family,
- your child's educators,
- your child's educational support staff,
- your child's behavioral support staff,
- school bus or school van drivers,
- cafeteria staff,
- school nurse, and
- school administrators (principal, vice principal).

This list is not all inclusive, and certainly doesn't mean that these individuals *should* discipline your child; but they may be in a position to need rules, guidelines, and parameters set by you in order to contain, manage, and interpret a situation in which your child is involved. You will wish to be clear in communicating to the preceding list of individuals a protocol on which you are in agreement with, especially if it differs from the manner in which other same-aged children are treated for behaving in similar ways. In an educational setting, this should be documented with signatures confirming agreement.

What do I do if I disagree with the way my spouse or my in-laws discipline my child?

Address the situation promptly if you disagree or are uncomfortable with the way in which your spouse or family relations discipline your child with autism. Consistency is key in disciplining your child; mixed or crossed signals with regard to methods, approaches, and what is allowed and disallowed will convey confusion and uncertainty to your child (which could make things even more problematic).

Prevention instead of intervention is paramount here, too. Clearly communicate your expectations—what is acceptable and what is not—to anyone who has the potential to discipline your child *before* such a situation arises. Otherwise you may find yourself struggling to put out fires as you go along, which only exacerbates your angst *and* the hurt feelings of those family members who thought they were doing the right thing *sans* your instruction. It is unfair to expect others to anticipate or infer how you would handle a given situation; be concise and direct in explaining your rationale for disciplining in the manner that you'd like to see based on what you've been learning about autism.

How do I communicate my expectations to my child with autism?

As a parent, you have the right to hold the same expectations of your child with autism as you would for any of your other children, regardless of how significantly compromised your child with autism appears to be. The difference lies in *how* you communicate your parental expectations.

As you have come to understand, it is important to reinforce your spoken words wherever possible with visuals such as written words paired with pictures, but especially to convey concepts you wish your child to retain. In the spirit of prevention instead of intervention, you should convey your expectations *prior* to requesting that your child act on them. You may reinforce these expectations through gentle reminders, practice, and praise for success as you would for any child.

For example, if you expect your child to clear her breakfast dishes from the table and place them in the sink, you should show her how to do so immediately following the two of you finishing a bowl of breakfast cereal. Let your child know she is big enough to take her dishes to the sink on her own, just like you do. Show her how you would like it done, and ask that she do the same. A written and pictorial narrative explaining this sequence in simple steps will reiterate the process and make it concrete when you read it with your child before this task. (Bear in mind that your approach may need fine-tuning. For instance, state clearly that the cereal bowl gets placed *gently* into the sink.) You may fade the amount of prompting as your child becomes increasingly independent and demonstrates that she understands the task. If you establish a picture schedule or chore chart in your home, this task may be added to it with the parental expectation that your child will now follow through.

How do I determine consequences for my child's behavior?

To determine consequences for your child's behavior, focus on teaching three principles that should resonate for a child with autism: cause and effect, natural consequences, and personal responsibility for one's actions. Cause and effect is the result of your child not acting on the expectations you have set forth (as long as you believe you've clearly communicated those expectations), the after-effect of which is something not intended. Not every circumstance can be anticipated, but instilling these principles in your child at a young age will hold lifelong value.

Staying with the previous example of clearing breakfast dishes, if your child opts not to gently place the bowl in the sink but instead tosses it, missing the sink and making a mess on the floor, the cause and effect is that if you do not place your bowl gently into the sink, it may spill to the floor and create a mess. The natural consequence of deliberately engaging in this action after you, the parent, has instructed your child how to clear dishes properly is that you will be angry or upset that (1) your child chose not to follow directions, and (2) your child has created a mess. Personal responsibility involves teaching your child to take ownership of her mistakes and do what she must to correct the situation and make it right. In this instance, that involves cleaning up the mess by placing the bowl into the kitchen sink the way your child knows she should, wiping up the mess, and disposing of it.

What is an appropriate way to discipline my child with autism?

Your child's autism diagnosis does not exempt him from parental discipline. As long as you have approached the prospect of discipline fairly and with compassionate accommodation, you may consider disciplining your child with autism in the same ways that you would discipline any of your children, using any of the myriad parenting techniques and strategies available from other sources.

Appropriate ways to discipline may include the following:

- Give the child a fair warning. For example, visually show your child the limitations he is creating by counting while holding up your fingers; indicate his progressive deterioration with a pictorial check mark, a "frowny" face (as opposed to a smiley face) sticker, or any other *visual and sequential* method.

- Communicate natural consequences if your child persists (which would entail what you have determined as punishment) using "if–then" language paired with visual prompts. For example: "Do not throw your bowl (point to bowl). Your bowl belongs in the sink (point to sink). *If* you throw your bowl again, *then* _____ will happen."
- Use time out. (Although many parents report that sending a child with autism to his room is not viewed as "punishment" by the child; so time out might instead consist of requesting that your child stay seated within your view.)
- Take away a privilege. (This may include an added or special "extra" related to your child's passion but *not* withholding your child's passion in its entirety.)
- Ground the child; that is, do not allow any activities—especially favored opportunities—outside of the home for a specified duration of time.

As the parent imposing discipline, you have a plan in mind with regard to duration. Your child with autism does not know this *unless* you have communicated it. Your child's concept of duration time may be vague or nonexistent. It is a fair and compassionate accommodation to be clear in communicating the duration of time of the punishment by visually showing your child on a calendar, on a clock, or—better yet—on a ticking kitchen timer.

Is spanking an appropriate way to discipline my child with autism?

Remember that your child with autism is inherently gentle and exquisitely sensitive. Recall, too, the chapter on mental health issues (Chapter 6) and the discussion on post-traumatic stress disorder. Striking or spanking your child may send a very strong message about who is in charge—but is it the proper message, and are you prepared for the potential long-term consequences? These may include your child's increasing withdrawal from you or that he may feel justified in hitting back in the throes of a meltdown because you have taught that hitting is acceptable.

You may be surprised to know that firm and consistent discipline has a far greater impact than spanking ever could. Still, you are a human being, and human beings say and do things in the heat of the moment that they later regret. One mom learned through trial and error after she "lost it" and raised her voice: "We try not to dwell on negatives or yell. I think yelling at a child with hypersensitive hearing is as tough on them as if you had spanked them." If you have acted on impulse or in haste and you recognize and regret it, you can always make it better by sincerely apologizing to your child and pledging to do better.

How do I deal with my other kids thinking my child with autism is being given special treatment?

As far as discipline is concerned, your other children will be less likely to think you are giving your child with autism "special treatment" if there *is* no special treatment. Aside from the explanations for understanding how your child may best think and process information so that you can discipline fairly, there is no reason why you can't implement the recommendations made here for *all* of your children, in whole, part, or in conjunction with other methods. In particular, all of your children may benefit from the clear, deliberate, and visual approach you may use with your child with autism. With the entire family on the same discipline plan, your job as a parent is easier (you don't have to remember special rules) and you will be able to consistently demonstrate that everyone is held to the same expectations, consequences, and disciplinary actions.

My child with autism talks and tries giving me lengthy explanations when I'm disciplining her—how do I deal with this?

If your child is trying to give you a lengthy explanation during your disciplinary measures, then it is probably time to back up and consider whether you may have jumped the gun or acted unfairly. Accidents happens, and mistakes occur; and a child who talks is entitled to present her side of the story in order to plead her case for leniency *prior to* any applied discipline on your part. You may be astonished to learn that it is *you* who has completely misinterpreted the situation at hand on learning of your child's explanation—which may be the polar opposite from your initial perception. Or, on hearing your child's rationale, you may grant some latitude based on your child's genuine misunderstanding of certain circumstances—which may have lead her to "overcorrect" a situation in trying to do the right thing, which, in turn, made things worse.

Finally, thank goodness you have a child with autism who has the ability to speak and can offer you an explanation of her behavior so that your role as a parent involves far less second-guessing in decoding your child's conduct and actions.

Should I discipline my speaking child if I ask him to give me an explanation for something that happened and he won't say anything?

Even the child with autism who talks may be unable to fully and completely articulate his position on his involvement in an incident of some sort without feeling overwhelming emotions of despair, distress, and anxiety. You should consider this premise first, if your initial inclination is to assume that your child with autism is being deliberately deceptive. Most kids tell untruths, some more than others, but it is unusual for someone with autism not to be forthcoming in saying what he means and meaning what he says.

Respect that your child may need some process time to acclimate himself to what's transpired in order to make sense of the situation and report it in a way that reflects his truth. One compassionate accommodation you can make is to request that your child provide his explanation to you in writing. Many of us better express our experiences and thoughts using the written word, and you can do this by asking your child to handwrite or type his answer to you. In fact, if your child is computer savvy and uses email, you can usually reach him and get a thorough and truthful answer by sending him an electronic communication, as opposed to having a direct one-on-one confrontation.

What can I do if my child's sense of justice and injustice seems very black and white and rigid?

Deconstructing your child's unyielding sense of what is right and what is wrong is likely to be an ongoing process that has the potential to endure into adulthood, because it can be a very difficult concept for some people on the autism spectrum to integrate. It is like driving a car: everyone knows the rules (otherwise they wouldn't have been granted a license), but that doesn't mean everyone follows them consistently—people break the speed limit, make U-turns where they shouldn't, and run red lights. Many of us have been guilty of one of these offenses at some time or another, but that shouldn't forever color the manner in which we are perceived by others. The child with autism, however, may brand such an individual as a lawbreaker. Your child's rigid sense of justice and injustice may make him unpopular with his peers if he is considered a "whistle-blower" or tattletale who reports every minor infraction. One young boy, who turned in classmates who weren't using the swing set safely, said it was his civic duty to report them.

This concept may create conflict when you attempt to discipline the child who is in error but feels justified in maintaining his position. One of the most compelling ways to educate your child with regard to making concessions and allowing some latitude is to always seek to relate the circumstances at hand back to a similar situation in which your child did something he shouldn't have, and didn't like it when someone else told on him. By making the situation an analogy (analogies are often successful for people with autism, who can fail to grasp the context of a situation), you've personalized an impersonal circumstance. For example, using the swing set scenario, you might counsel your child by being remindful of the time he jumped from the monkey bars when it was against the rules to do so—elicit his perspective on how it would've felt if someone had turned him in for misusing playground equipment in the same way, despite the fact that he may have had good reasons. (Using this strategy doesn't mean your child's going to like it, but it's a good way to analyze cause and effect.)

If your child remains inflexible, compose a written narrative with him, like those at the end of this book, in which degrees of urgency that do or do not require reporting are discussed. Thoughts include assessing whether someone is at risk of being harmed, and whether or not there is a nearby authority figure to mediate the situation. Natural consequences might include your child being branded a tattletale or experiencing abandoned friendships. A strong code of ethics is nothing to be ashamed of; encourage your child to weigh the options and adopt an aptitude for flexibility. This is a process that will take time, practice, and real-life experience.

How do I deal with it if my child tries applying his discipline rules to me and his siblings?

You are your child's parent, and you set the tone for what will and will not be tolerated with regard to disrespect of your parental obligation to discipline (i.e., teach) your child right from wrong. However, unless you believe your child's behavior is purely retaliatory (and you've been cautioned about jumping to those conclusions where autism is concerned), do not misconstrue it as being without purpose. It may well be a communication expressed in the one way your child understands to express it herself. That is, in attempting to impose rules of discipline on you, is your child really identifying a flawed system in which she has no say in communicating her displeasure with *your* behavior?

As your child's parent, you are the adult in charge; but you are also a human being who makes mistakes on a daily basis. Parenting can be a dynamic, trial-and-error process full of faults and pitfalls. You will make misjudgments that may cause your child to react with strong opposition. Can you see past the affront you may feel from the child who appears to be trying to turn the tables on you but is, in reality, objecting to your parenting style in the moment? If so, take some quiet time to model appropriate conduct by honestly confessing your shortcomings and pledging to correct your mistake. This doesn't mean you abandon your rules for discipline, nor should you allow your child to continue "disciplining" you or your other children. But by being open and honest, you will establish a tone of fair compromise in the two-way relationship that is parent and child.

Am I wrong to tolerate my child pulling my hair or scratching me when I'm attempting to discipline her?

Would you tolerate any of your *undiagnosed* children pulling your hair or scratching you during disciplinary measures? By allowing your child with autism to perpetuate this conduct, you are sending a message that condones and coddles your child because she is "special," and that the regular rules of parental expectation don't apply because she has autism. This kind of overprotective stance is a disservice to your child that, in time, may make things worse as she grows and matures and potentially reacts with intensified aggression.

Make clear your objection to this improper conduct in ways your child will best understand; remain firm and, if necessary, apply the disciplinary procedures previously outlined if your child breaches the code you have set forth. This doesn't dismiss your child's actions of pulling hair or scratching as noncommunications—clearly they are communicating *something*, ranging from displeasure to fear to anxiety. In fact, this kind of conduct may manifest itself more in the child who does not speak. Acknowledge that your child is upset, attempt to discern its source, and then suggest she express it in another, more functional outlet such as physical activity, drawing, singing, or role-playing with toys. Affirm that she doesn't have to like the way you discipline, but those are the rules and you expect her to abide by them.

Do I discipline if my child melts down when one of my other children plays loud music, but he goes into his bedroom and plays music just as loudly?

At this point in your reading, you are in a position to better understand the degrees with which your child likely experiences his sensory sensitivities and the rationale for the apparent paradox of your child's loud music versus the loud music of another. In making compassionate accommodations for your child's sensory sensitivities, you should establish household rules about tolerable noise levels for everyone. This means that no one should play loud music (beyond a level everyone agrees on) if others in the house are likely to be affected by it—unable to think, read, communicate, engage in another activity, or concentrate.

If you have established this rule and someone breaks it, and your child with autism has a strong reaction, it would be unfair to punish him for responding to the unpredictable overstimulation. By the same token, you should apply disciplinary measures if your child with autism imposes the same inconsideration on others by disregarding the rule set for acceptable noise level. To avoid any confusion or debate, ensure that the maximum level allowed for noise is conveyed visually in writing and/or with a colored sticker or magic marker dot on everyone's music devices.

How do I handle it when my child keeps running out of the house unattended?

Running out of the house unattended and seemingly heedless of danger (formally called *elopement*) is a serious issue for obvious reasons, but it is a common experience for parents plagued by the impulsivity of the child who, at a moment's notice, bolts unexpectedly. As a result, many parents have installed outdoor fencing, locks strategically placed as high as possible, alarms on doors and windows, and have even equipped their children with commercially manufactured tracking devices—and still some children manage to elude like Houdini. These may sound like extreme measures, but elopement is not to be taken lightly; the media regularly reports on children with autism who go missing, and who may or may not be recovered safely after wandering off.

This is yet another situation of prevention instead of intervention. The implications of running away unattended are apparent to you, but not necessarily so to your child with autism. Suffice it to say, your child's elopement is a communication of something. It may be as simple as a natural curiosity about exploring his neighborhood, or it may be as complex as escaping an unbearable situation. One adult woman with autism reflected on the times she ran out into the street in front of moving cars; as a child, she rationalized that the cars would simply see her and stop moving in order to make way. To curtail your child's desire to run away, you'll need to be very clear in communicating the following:

- Set parameters in ways that are visual and concrete. (To start, a written narrative explaining trespassing, found at the back of this book, may be adapted as a template.)
- Your child should be shown the physical boundaries of his own living area (including any yard space), and should be instructed never to cross those boundaries without adult supervision.
- Provide your child with a way to convey her desire to go out of doors, and provide clear-cut and visual indicators as to when you can fulfill that request.
- Discuss the dangerous impact of being hit by a car, drowning, being kidnapped, or becoming lost—not to frighten or threaten, but within the context of natural consequences.
- Enforce disciplinary measures if your child breaches the agreed-on rules.
- Regularly review the rules until you are certain your child comprehends and obeys.

Do I discipline my five-year-old child with autism any differently than my eleven-year-old with autism?

Consistency in parental discipline—and sticking to it—is going to be important for the child with autism regardless of age. This is key. Households in which children (whether they have autism or not) are out of control are frequently loud and chaotic environments with no structure or routine in place. When parenting a child with autism, it is not helpful to make up the rules as you go along, flying by the seat of your pants, so to speak. Don't set you and your children up for failure by reaping what you sow—in this instance, a bitter harvest. Instead, focus on consistency within the context of this book's themes: presumption of intellect, prevention instead of intervention, fostering self-advocacy, and the recognition of "behaviors" as functional attempts to communicate. (Remember, too, that your children with autism may be quick to highlight lapses in consistency from one to another in terms of discipline.) Bearing these concepts in mind will benefit your family of more than one child with autism despite differences in age, and will guide you in making judgment calls in instances of parental latitude for either of your children.

How do I handle it when I'm accused of being the only one who knows how to manage my child?

The operative word in this question is *accused*, which implies that the persons with whom you and your child with autism interact are jealous, impatient, or possibly resentful of your ability to support your child so that she feels safe and comfortable and in control. As was true of deciding to educate family members about your child's autism, determine if it is appropriate or in your child's best interest to communicate the tenets and ideals you have been learning in order to successfully embrace your child's autism with those who are making you feel affronted.

You can approach this situation with indifference and offense, or you can see it as an opportunity to advocate on your child's behalf. If you choose the latter, try re-envisioning your role as parent to a child with autism as that of an ambassador of goodwill and an agent of change in a global effort to transform hurt feelings, insensitivity, even prejudice in those who misunderstand your child's unique way of being. If this book has inspired you in some small measure, you can create a ripple effect of change—one person at a time—through your demonstration of courtesy and respect for your child in the presence of others.

What do I do when I have been asked not to attend my place of religion due to my child's behaviors?

Being asked not to attend your place of religion because of your child's *behaviors* is not the same as being asked not to attend because of your child's *autism*. Before taking further action, find a contact in your place of worship who is in a position to clarify the circumstances. Listen carefully, present your impressions, affirm your commitment to include your child, and be prepared to offer solutions. On the surface, it may seem as though your religion is preaching one thing and practicing another by seeking to exclude your child. Indeed, this is likely the case in some instances; as a society we are slowly improving the ways in which we publicly accommodate persons with *physical* disabilities, but we are a long way from similarly supporting persons with "invisible" disabilities, such as autism spectrum experiences that can be interpreted as purely behavioral.

If this is truly an issue of your child having been disruptive continuously and severely enough to be asked not to attend religious service, what are the preventive measures you can take in order to keep your child involved? Is there an autism-specific educational opportunity present? In what ways can you offer your child strategies and incentives to participate in part or in whole? Is there alternative programming in which your child, and other children, may participate? How can the environment be adapted, or how can your child's sensory sensitivities best be accommodated? What occurs before, during, and after service that might create an adverse reaction in your child?

Perhaps more so than any other environment, the attending patrons of your place of worship have the right to attend service with the expectation that everyone in attendance respects unwritten rules of common courtesy in observance of solitude and contemplation—that is not an unreasonable expectation. Your role as a parent is to balance upholding this philosophy with including your child with autism as a participant

What is the "dignity of risk"?

As the parent of a child with unique abilities that so often get misinterpreted and misunderstood, you naturally wish to protect your child from being labeled as inferior or maligned for her differences. This means that you may find yourself intercepting, interceding, and struggling to determine how best to insulate your child from outcomes that may have any kind of negative ramifications for her. Remember a reference to the idea of "learned helplessness" in the Treatment Options chapter (Chapter 8) under "What causes some children to regress in their skills?" While your endeavor is admirable and altruistic, borne of parental love, please know that you are ultimately temporary in your child's life, as harsh as that may sound. The big world is full of letdowns, disappointments, and hard feelings. By constantly micromanaging your child's life, are you creating an artificial insulation that is inevitably more a disservice than a service?

Disciplining your child should be a teaching and learning opportunity about making decisions and choices. The "dignity of risk" pertains to those natural learning opportunities by which you exercise restraint (which may be very challenging) in order for your child to grow by understanding the repercussions of his actions. This doesn't mean you stand by and watch your child enter into harm's way—you would, and should, most assuredly intervene! The dignity of risk calls for providing your child with the chance to make short- and long-term mistakes, accept responsibility for her actions, and enjoy follow-up counsel with you in order to process what has transpired. In other words, allow minor opportunities for your child to make decisions and choices you wouldn't have advised in order for her to grow and learn from her mistakes.

This does not mean that you withhold discipline. The dignity of risk requires you to focus on the issue, not the person. When your child makes mistakes, assure her that she is still loved and valued but also discuss consequences for her actions in addition to a dialogue about making good, better, and best choices the next time a similar situation presents itself. (Remember that your child with autism likely retains information via a strong associative link in the moment.) Teaching the dignity of risk emphasizes the development of self-discipline instead of parental discipline.

At what point will my child stop needing to be disciplined?

The answer to this question has more to do with semantics than it does with believing your child with autism will forever be dependent on you for parental discipline. Your child may always look on you as a source of loving guidance and support in navigating life in all its unpredictability, in the same way you may seek the intimate counsel of a parent, sibling, or family member who knows you well and will see you through. How you provide that guidance and support depends on your parenting style.

Providing persistent discipline in ways that are punitive (i.e., using a tough-love approach) will probably only alienate your very sensitive child as he grows and matures. Allowing him the independence to assert himself through developing self-discipline (the dignity of risk), combined with the reliability of your loving presence, makes for a relationship that can segue from a parent–child relationship to a peer partnership as your child grows to adulthood. In this way, your support will slowly transform into that of advisement and counsel.

Chapter 10

MAKING SOCIAL CONNECTIONS

- Why won't my speaking child ever say "I love you" to me?
- My child has no interest in making friends with other children—how do I handle this?
- What do I do when people think my child is simply overly shy and withdrawn?
- Am I wrong to push my child to have lots of friends?
- Is it okay to tell my child's friends about his autism?
- How do I teach my child to recognize communications such as irony or sarcasm?
- How do I help my child learn to identify the emotions she's feeling? At times she is visibly upset, crying, or anxious, yet she can't explain what she is upset about.
- How do I handle it if my son has a tendency to talk too much and it turns other kids off?
- How can I get my child to stop talking to himself, especially in front of others?
- What do I do if my child is socially isolating himself because he chews on his shirt or his pencil and gets saliva everywhere?
- How come my child seems to interact with others better on the computer?
- How come my child wants to talk with adults but not kids her own age?
- How do I get my child to understand that pretending to be a dinosaur on the recess playground scares away other kids who might otherwise be friendly?
- I'm told that in the cafeteria, my child doesn't interact with kids at his table—why not?
- How do I help my child when he interrupts others constantly?
- Should I teach my child to ask clarifying questions if she doesn't understand something? Won't she stick out?
- What is *movie talk* or *scripting*?
- What if it seems like my child thinks he is a cartoon character most of the time?
- How can movie talk be practically applied?
- My daughter with autism kissed a boy older than she is because he said he'd give her money—how do I get her to understand the concept of ulterior motives?
- Can adults take advantage of my child because he doesn't question what people tell him and believes they're telling the truth?
- My child is well liked by his Little League team, but now that he's middle school-aged, I'm starting to see him become more frustrated with his own physical limitations—how do I handle this?

- How can I help my child see that the world isn't always fair, and sometimes people do things we don't expect?
- How do I help my teen with autism who has a couple of close friends, but lately doesn't want to spend time with them?
- My teenage son is extremely moral. How do I help him understand when he gets socially isolated because he "tells" on his male peers when they start talking about sex, scantily clad girls, porn, etc.?
- My teen with autism has never had a romantic attachment, and says she doesn't care to. Should I believe her, and is this a problem?
- My child has a romantic crush on a girl that is not welcomed, and he has been discouraged by her. How do I help him understand this rejection when he insists she likes him?

Why won't my speaking child ever say "I love you" to me?

Like shaking hands and making eye contact in conversation, certain social reciprocations need to be taught—even if we don't feel them in the moment. (For instance, have you ever responded with "Fine" when someone asks you how you are, even if you're feeling lousy?) The trouble is, unlike handshaking and eye contact, love is intangible, and will require an explanation that includes equating love with affectionate tangibles like soft, soothing words, embraces and gentle touching, and pleasurable time together united in an activity or event that creates great joy and happiness. Your child with autism who speaks may need to be taught that when someone close to her says the words "I love you," it is usually expected to respond in kind or at least to acknowledge the sentiment. You will need to explain to her that there are times when people expect to hear "I love you" because it makes them feel good inside.

Even if your child knows to reply by rote, she may be unaware of independently initiating verbal expressions of love, and that there is no limit to the number of times one can communicate love. For example, one mom was so dismayed that her son with autism never said "I love you" that she confronted him about it. At seven years old, he very matter of factly reminded her that he had indeed said that he loved her—four years prior when he was three! In his way of thinking, the boy believed saying "I love you" once established it as fact from that time forward, and anything more was superfluous.

But aren't there other ways in which children with autism who speak—and those that do not—express their love without knowing to say it? Pay close attention to those out-of-the-blue, unexpected moments in which your child surprises you with a thoughtful gesture, a piece of artwork, or a loving hug. Be prepared to acknowledge those actions as communications, and convey your gratitude for your child's expression of love and affection. This may also be a time to practice reciprocating the communication of "I love you" in whatever manner your child feels comfortable (and remember that Eskimos say "I love you" by rubbing noses together).

My child has no interest in making friends with other children—how do I handle this?

You might better qualify your question by rephrasing it in the following way: "My child *appears to have* no interest in making friends..." Even though autism spectrum clinical criteria call for someone to favor isolated, intrinsic activities over social interactions, that does not mean it holds true for everyone. Many adult self-advocates have expressed their desperate desire to connect socially with others in order to have a sense of community, friendship, and belonging. The challenge lies in being perceived as unusual or different. Your child may not know what to say or say too much, coupled with autistic features that may be interpreted as idiosyncratic (or just plain weird), which often leads to social ostracism in no uncertain terms.

You should also reflect on the opportunities you child has had previously for such interactions—did she succeed? If not, or if your child has had very unpleasant, unfriendly experiences with others, it could be that she feels no incentive because she has suffered emotional distress. If that has happened, for some it is easier to simply withdraw and not make the effort. As a starting point to offer your child the chance to expand socially, please revisit the chapter on valuing passions (Chapter 7). Consider how to support your child to begin making those initial connections with children her age that share similar interests.

What do I do when people think my child is simply overly shy and withdrawn?

You are bound to meet some people who are judgmental and not particular about speaking their mind when confronted by anything or anyone who challenges their perception of "the norm." In telling you your child with autism is too shy and withdrawn, they are probably comparing your child against their own children, or those children of others, who are thought to be "typical" kids and far more socially adept.

When this occurs, you can choose to ignore the remark, or you can choose to buffer it in a way that will effectively diffuse any deliberate intent. If you opt for the latter, try replying with a proud and beaming smile and saying something like "Bill is quiet because he spends so much time deep in thought—he's always creating or making plans for something great" or "Jessica is just really gentle in her own sweet way, and we adore her for it." You should not, though, feel at all obligated to disclose your child's autism diagnosis to persons who make such casual remarks—nor should you do so without your child's prior consent (appropriately obtained beginning at whatever age it is you have revealed your child's diagnosis to her).

Am I wrong to push my child to have lots of friends?

There's a difference between providing natural opportunities to develop social connections that may lead to friendships and pressing your child to create artificial relationships because it seems "normal." By pushing your child with autism to have lots of friends, do you mean by force or, at the least, strong expectation? If so, you may be making things worse by creating discomfort and anxiety for your child and leading him to feel disinterested, unprepared, and unwilling to emulate popular conceptions of having lots of friends.

Remember, it only takes one good friend—one stalwart ally—to have a comfortable, reliable, and mutually pleasing relationship. This may be difficult to accept if you are someone who values having many social contacts, chatting on the phone, going to parties, and making lunch dates. Acknowledge that your child with autism is not a social butterfly, may never be a social butterfly—and maybe doesn't want to be. A lasting friendship is going to be the one your child chooses to enjoin because he *wants* to, not because he *has* to. In the interim, continue exploring natural opportunities for your child to engage with others through mutual likes, interests, and passions.

Is it okay to tell my child's friends about his autism?

It is never okay to disclose your child's autism diagnosis without his permission, any more than you'd want him running around the neighborhood disclosing personal attributes you'd prefer not be broadcast about yourself—it is no one's business, and no one needs to know. If you're posing this inquiry, it may be because the ways in which your child thinks, interacts, and interprets social processes has come into question or created potentially problematic situations.

To affect some measure of resolve, you should enact the preventive measure of teaching him to deconstruct social situations, or counsel him in appropriate ways to communicate his distress or discomfort to other children. Partner with him to decide what kinds of information would be helpful to know in advance of similar situations in order to decode what is happening. Determine if your child requires your further assistance, or if there is a way you can aid him in communicating to his friends by role-playing, scripting what to say beforehand, or self-advocating certain needs by way of clarifying or explaining to the other children. And remember that all kids argue, fight, and make up regardless of diagnosis.

How do I teach my child to recognize communications such as irony or sarcasm?

As referenced earlier in the chapter on communication, understanding sarcasm, irony, innuendo, double-entendre, and slang is natural for people who are "typical." It would seem that most people seamlessly assimilate these concepts through osmosis, by virtue of growing up and leading fairly usual and social lives. However, for the child on the autism spectrum who interprets everything so literally, these commonplace idioms are like trying to crack a secret code—one that everyone else seems privy to.

Remember the story of *Alice in Wonderland?* In that book, Alice was the "typical" individual trying to socially integrate with others in a foreign world, one that somewhat paralleled the world from which she'd been displaced, but one that came with lots of social misunderstanding and misinterpretations. As far as the inhabitants of Wonderland were concerned, Alice might as well have been autistic! To Alice, the characters she encountered spoke in rhymes and riddles and nonsense, but their way of being had a logic that made sense to them. Also, Alice had no real friends or allies. Instead she was confronted by characters who were harsh, abrasive, insensitive, and intolerant of her perceived shortcomings as she struggled to fit in and make sense of their nonsense. In real life, your child may be a lot like Alice.

An earlier example given when discussing communication was about "shaking a leg." Other common slips of the tongue that may need deciphering include:

- He lost his head (or marbles).
- Mix by hand.
- Duck!
- That's cool.

- She has to eat crow.
- Get lost!
- Don't beat a dead horse.
- You've got ants in your pants.
- I've got egg on my face.
- He's green with envy.
- That's to die for!
- I'm getting a little hoarse (horse).
- She broke my heart.

As you can see, these social idioms are woven throughout our everyday language but have the potential to be taken completely out of context if interpreted literally. Your child will require your sensitive and patient explanations, in ways he'll best understand, to crack the secret code. Until your child masters the code, don't be surprised if you find yourself having a debriefing session on a regular, if not daily, basis.

How do I help my child learn to identify the emotions she's feeling? At times she is visibly upset, crying, or anxious, yet she can't explain what she is upset about.

When your child is upset, crying, or anxious, she may not be in a position to put words to what she is feeling in the moment because it is overwhelming her. This kind of internal, cataclysmic confusion is common in persons with autism who are extremely sensitive and easily overwrought. Were you ever so frightened or angered that words escaped you? Have you ever had a crying jag in which it was hard to catch your breath and difficult to articulately express what was wrong? It may be the same for the child with autism who is overcome—except the response is magnified. In the moment, try the following:

- Offer quiet process time for your child to decompress and make sense of jumbled thoughts.
- Try just holding her without saying anything.
- Recommend your child waylay her focus by engaging in her self-soothing activity until she calms.
- Ask your child to sing, draw, write, or type her impressions.
- Offer gentle, soothing words or music to help quell her upset mood.

Outside of those moments of extreme emotion, you will want to practice identifying and communicating emotions in ways that are visual. It's no coincidence that many young children with autism are drawn to *Thomas the Tank Engine*; aside from being more tolerable to gaze on than a human face, the very pronounced facial features of the anthropomorphic Thomas characters make abundantly clear their emotions. You can work with your child to identify feelings and emotions in similar ways by deconstructing the Sunday comics, favorite cartoon or movie scenes, or characters in video games. Supporting your child to define these emotions in a pleasing way outside of the time when they need to be used may aid her in putting a name to her feelings when it is needed most.

How do I handle it if my son has a tendency to talk too much and it turns other kids off?

The tendency for some children with autism to focus on a particular subject of passion and talk it into the ground, so to speak, is common in those who communicate verbally and are unsure of social parameters. (It is also the hallmark of one who is trying to engage socially and wishes to be acknowledged for his talents.) Here is another example of needing to prepare in advance by equipping your child with knowledge of the ebbs and flows of conversation. There are a variety of ways to approach this.

You may wish to encourage your child to create, through drawing or computer art, a typical conversation between friends and acquaintances, complete with overlapping dialogue balloons in order to illustrate what happens whenever one person dominates the conversation instead of taking turns. Taking turns may be delineated by stating only two or three sentences at a time, and pausing before awaiting a response. If someone changes the subject, that's a social indication of disinterest or desire to discuss something new that should be respected.

You may also practice conversations by role-playing and coaching your child. This may include teaching subtle indicators that someone is becoming bored or impatient such as rolling their eyes, looking at their watch, tapping their foot, rolling their hands to show "hurry up," or making an exasperated sigh. With your child's permission, you may videotape him informally and, in private, gently process his impressions with him when watching the playback—this can be quite revealing as we tend to see ourselves differently than others see us.

Understanding verbal social interactions is like ordering from a menu; you don't tell the waitress your life story, you just give her enough information to get you what you want. Practicing, rehearsing, role-playing, and illustration are sound ways to take authorship for composing one's own menu selections.

How can I get my child to stop talking to himself, especially in front of others?

Your child may or may not even realize he is talking out loud to himself, and could be unaware that it is leading to a social stigma. Many of us talk to ourselves out loud, especially to aid us in thinking through an emotional process or to complete a sequence of activities mentally tallied. Where your child with autism is concerned, there may be several reasons for talking to himself:

- The additional input of verbalizing an activity may serve to help him to focus on the task at hand.
- He may be using his verbalizations as a self-soothing technique to reduce anxiety in the moment.
- If his voice level is elevated, he might be blocking out painful, external auditory stimuli.
- He may be talking his body through certain motoric movements that are challenging to enact.
- He may be verbally replaying an event that created confusion, upset, or trauma.
- He may be feeling bored and unchallenged, and is amusing himself by repeating a movie, cartoon, or video game he's seen.

Paying careful attention to what your child is saying may aid in deciphering why he's doing it and how to curb it in social settings. If you feel strongly that your child's talking to himself in front of others is detrimental, privately, gently, and respectfully coach him into learning how to reduce his speech to a whisper under his breath, or to mentally speak the words in silence.

What do I do if my child is socially isolating himself because he chews on his shirt or his pencil and gets saliva everywhere?

Bear in mind that your child has good reasons for doing what he's doing, and he's doing the best he knows how to; your child is not intending to deliberately isolate himself socially. If your child is on medication that causes dry mouth as a side effect (which many meds do), he may be trying to work up some saliva if water fountain breaks are not frequent enough. Oftentimes the need for someone with autism to chew on something may be linked to a requirement for oral stimulation and input.

The rhythm of repeated chewing accelerates the heartbeat, blood pressure, and blood flow to the brain by at least 25 percent—enough to awaken the left and right hemispheres of the brain in order for both to align or "entrain" in synchronization. Recent studies have indicated that chewing gum can relieve stress, increase attentiveness, boost concentration, and aid in accessing memory. It may be that your child engages in frequent chewing because it feels good in his mouth and keeps him alert!

If gum chewing is allowed in your child's school, ensure that he has a supply of sugarless and pleasant-tasting (not overwhelming) gum accessible throughout the day. For obvious reasons, bubble gum is not recommended, but a hard gum that requires lots of jaw power to soften may work best. Educate your child in "gum etiquette"—no cracking or popping, chewing with your mouth closed, and appropriate disposal when finished. Your child may no longer need to chew gum if he spits it out or starts to play with it (at which time, the point about appropriate disposal should be reinforced).

If gum chewing is not allowed in your child's school, but you can get a doctor, occupational therapist, or other professional to recommend it, you can require that gum chewing be a documented educational accommodation to meet your child's needs during the day. Gum chewing keeps your child's saliva flowing (which can offset medicinal side effects) and keeps the saliva in his mouth, which is the desirable alternative to getting his shirt wet or chewing on a pencil. Best of all, nearly all kids chew gum, and in so doing, your child will avert the social stigmatization that may be the cause of your concern.

How come my child seems to interact with others better on the computer?

Your child with autism seems to interact better with others over the computer for the same reason that it is challenging for her to hold a thoughtful, intelligent conversation face to face and maintain direct eye contact. (Revisit Chapter 3 for more information on communication.) Please do not perceive this as a sign of social impairment; communicating with others over the computer *is* social!

In particular, your child may better relate to others via computer technology because it is absent the awkwardness and distracting visuals of in-person dialogue. Have you discovered that when you really want to communicate your thoughts in a comprehensive way, you express yourself better in writing? The same holds true for many people on the autism spectrum for whom real-time social interactions prove challenging. If your child emails with others, she can respond to the message in her own time, thoughtfully, and without the social expectations of immediate response. Lots of young people use "emoticons" when emailing and instant messaging—small "smiley face" style icons that visually convey, in shorthand, a wide variety of feelings in response and reaction to online exchanges. This may not only cut down on misinterpretations for the context of written communications, it may also provide your child with a nonintrusive way to identify emotions and pair them with appropriate content.

Your child will best be poised to broaden social circles by connecting via the Internet with others who share her most passionate of interests. There are websites, chat rooms, message boards, and listserv groups to explore and partake in with the same cautions about using the Internet that the parent of any child would enact. By encouraging safe and pleasing online interactions, you may support your child in bridging social gaps.

How come my child wants to talk with adults but not kids her own age?

The child with autism who is drawn to converse more with adults than her peers may be significantly challenged in relating to her age group for several reasons. If your child is aware of her own social limitations, or is being made to feel different by her peers, then she likely also feels no incentive to engage with the very people she'd rather avoid! Determine if this is the case, and take swift action if your child is being bullied.

Many kids on the autism spectrum are experts in their field of passionate interest; and oftentimes those interests are so minute, selective, or advanced that only an adult might be as knowledgeable or intrigued as your child. If you are closely attentive, you may over-hear your child engaging in "inner-circle" banter with an adult comrade around a particular and unique topic of interest. Adults also tend to be more accepting and forgiving of diversity, and may be prone to indulge your child's interests, while her peers may, in no uncertain terms, be harshly critical or even ostracizing.

Please review Chapter 7, "Valuing Passions," for tips on connecting your child with peers who share the same areas of passion; but please also preserve your child's relationships with the adults in her life, as long as they are healthy relationships. As children, any number of us may have been positively inspired or duly influenced through the generosity of a sensitive and doting adult who nurtured and encouraged us into shaping our future. It would be a shame to see your child's relationships with adults extinguished solely because of her label, or because it is believed that maintaining such relation-ships is "inappropriate."

How do I get my child to understand that pretending to be a dinosaur on the recess playground scares away other kids who might otherwise be friendly?

First, let's acknowledge that your child who is pretending to be a dinosaur on the recess playground *is* trying to independently create social connections with his peers. He has good reasons for doing what he's doing, and he's doing the very best he knows how to in the moment with what he's got. Unless, in his reenactment, he's attacking, scratching, or biting others (which must be stopped immediately per school rules), he's just overshooting the mark by coming on a little too strong and off-putting potential friends. Fortunately, an interest in dinosaurs is a perennial favorite for lots of young kids, regardless of diagnosis, so there's a building block present from which to develop a sturdy foundation.

In addressing this circumstance, it would be helpful to partner with your child and his teacher, playground monitor, or educational support aide. Begin by asking your child to illustrate his interactions on the playground in order to help you understand it from his perspective. You now have something tangible from which to have a dialogue and begin to decode the misunderstanding. In ways that your child will best understand and retain, discuss the manner in which his social outreach is being interpreted by other children as threatening.

Your child is unlikely to yield at first because, after all, he's only behaving in the manner that the dinosaur he chose to emulate would behave (think *T. rex*). If this is the case, then the ensuing discussion should involve asking your child to list the friends his dinosaur would typically have. If there are none (because he's a predator), you might suggest that your child adopt the persona of a docile and benign dinosaur in order to better attract long-term playmates in the spirit of taking turns.

If he still refuses to yield, then he may be intentionally keeping others at a distance as opposed to just being confused. Given that case, your child will need adult intervention to provide structure to his play and that of potential friends to follow within the context of turn-taking and rules for good playground behavior. A preventive measure would involve an adult supervising the selection of dinosaur personas and a discussion of a scenario (with a beginning, middle, and end) to adhere to. If things get too intense, dinosaur play may need to be temporarily banned in favor of dinosaur discussions or structured dinosaur-themed games. Under adult facilitation, this situation requires gentle refining in order to keep things in check, avoid your child unwittingly isolating himself socially, and promote positive playground interactions.

I'm told that in the cafeteria, my child doesn't interact with kids at his table—why not?

Have you been in your child's cafeteria during lunchtime lately? It's a cacophony of overwhelming aromas and noises—everything from clanging silverware, dropped trays, and fever-pitch decibel levels of conversation to unpleasant food scents that may induce dizzying nausea in your child's sensory system. Your child may not be very social during lunchtime in the cafeteria because he's simply trying avoid becoming swallowed up by it all and totally losing it! (More on this is in Chapter 11, School Success.)

Like the preceding playground scenario, time spent in the cafeteria lunchroom is unstructured social time. It's seen as a social break for most kids, but for your child it's work—hard work at that. Trying to acclimate to the environment and pass for normal, or at least assimilate, may be very trying for the child with autism—and your child is expected to depart that environment and resume learning?

In what way can you advocate that compassionate accommodations be made for your child to encourage social connections? Do you know with whom he is paired at his lunch table—are they kids he knows and enjoys? Some schools use the "lunch bunch" approach by building on passions and seating kids who love to discuss the same things around the same table. This might require adult supervision and facilitation initially to get things jump-started by selecting a topic, or subtopic within a topic, to chat about over the meal. When successful, your child may be surprised to learn that he becomes so absorbed in conversation, he no longer hears the cafeteria din (or it's greatly diminished). This is a good strategy for offering social connections, and will look even more natural as soon as constant adult support is faded or made intermittent by the supervising adult visiting *all* lunchroom tables.

How do I help my child when he interrupts others constantly?

Many people—children and adults—on the autism spectrum interrupt others in conversation because they misinterpret the give and take of verbal communication. They may get so excited about the topic at hand that they end up walking on others' words. Or, they've heard enough of what they need to know from their communication partner and jump in before losing their train of thought. Perhaps you're the same way.

Your child's interrupting is not something that should be misconstrued as intentional—unless the concept has been taught and practiced. In fact, he may be completely unaware of it or that he's making a social faux pas and seems rude. In such a case, he requires you to privately, gently, and respectfully bring it to his attention in ways that he will best understand. Start by partnering with him to videotape or illustrate a common social interaction, each party playing the person who interrupts and the one interrupted. Debrief and process with your child how it feels to be both parties. During this process, you may learn more of your child's rationale for interrupting. Illustrate the manner in which conversation usually flows via turn-taking and waiting patiently for someone to finish speaking.

Explain how, when we interrupt, no one is clearly heard, and we are communicating to our partner that we don't value what they have to say because what we want to say is more important and takes priority. This can lead to confusion, misunderstandings, and hurt feelings. Your child is human, and will likely continue to interrupt at times; ensure that, as part of this process, you are teaching him to be conscious of catching himself instead of "hogging" the conversation (imagine that illustrated visual). Social faux pas are often forgiven with a sincere "Please forgive me." If your child feels it is absolutely urgent to interrupt, teach that it is acceptable to state "Please excuse me for interrupting, but … (your hair is on fire, for example!)."

Should I teach my child to ask clarifying questions if she doesn't understand something? Won't she stick out?

If your child doesn't understand what is being communicated to her (especially if it's a request or direction), there's absolutely nothing wrong with asking for the information to be repeated or restated another way. Some children with autism may "play deaf," appear incompetent, or agree to something they otherwise wouldn't do simply because they don't understand clearly what's been said, and they don't have the social tools to ask for clarity!

Teaching your child how to ask clarifying questions in order to ascertain the purpose and intent of a social communication is a tremendous strength. It is a building block toward independent self-advocacy that will be of lifelong good service to her. And who cares if it looks like she's sticking out—anyone who is worthy of your child will be more than happy to repeat or restate themselves in order to be clearly understood. As an adjunct, you may also wish to coach your child into writing it down, drawing it, or requesting that her communication partner do so, in order to fully process and absorb what's being said. Outside of a classroom setting, there's also nothing wrong with not responding to what's been said instantly, but instead replying with "Please let me think about this, and I'll get back to you with my answer."

What is *movie talk* or *scripting*?

The topic of *movie talk* or *scripting* that was alluded to in the Communication chapter (Chapter 3) will be more fully addressed here in the next several questions and answers. Children who are "typical" often learn to speak, enunciate, and read through repeatedly viewing or being read the same thing over and over—some seem to thrive on the repetition of a familiar story or video. Similarly, many children with autism are fascinated by—and rely on the consistency of—watching favorite movies, cartoons, commercials, and video games. Those same children may fall short in adequate social skills so they naturally compensate by "mimicking" lines of dialogue, emotional emphasis, and accompanying body language from characters they enjoy and admire. You may be truly amazed at the look-alike, sound-alike skill with which your child reproduces his movie talk. Oftentimes, the movie talk is employed functionally and appropriately; and, if you've been paying close attention, you'll be able to pinpoint the exact source of the dialogue your child is using in an effort to socially adapt. Such was the case for one stay-at-home mom whose daughter watched Disney's *Little Mermaid* video all day every day; when dad came home and scolded the girl for not picking up her toys, mom overhead (and instantly recognized) her daughter precisely enact Ariel the Mermaid's dialogue, "Father … no!"

What if it seems like my child thinks he is a cartoon character most of the time?

One of the myths about individuals with autism is that they are allegedly unable to imagine or engage in creative play as many children enjoy doing. Your child with autism does not think he's a cartoon character but if he's not feeling valued for his own identity, attributes, and talents, he may well align his identity more closely with that of the favored cartoon character to erect a façade that (in his thinking) others may find more acceptable, if not downright attractive. This may be cause for concern if children with autism spend more time projecting the persona of the cartoon character than they spend being themselves. The need for damage control should be obvious to the parent, who needs to reinforce that the child is loved and appreciated just as he is.

Another concern is if your child has adopted the dialogue and mannerisms of a destructive, villainous character (who are often portrayed as possessing a lot of control and magical powers). You should be able to recognize this, and your child will likely not discriminate where and with whom he opts to slip into this persona in order to communicate his desire to control a situation or keep others, who threaten to intrude, at a distance. Careful counseling in ways your child will best understand is necessary to prevent your child from undermining himself; start by visually reviewing sections of the movie or cartoon that feature the villain and discuss that character's motives, how that character is perceived by others, and how that character is, ultimately, punished or dispatched for injustices and misdeeds. Persuade your child to identify the positive attributes of more heroic characters and discuss or illustrate—and encourage—those desirable traits, especially when you see or hear your child beginning to demonstrate them uniquely.

How can movie talk be practically applied?

All too often, movie talk is perceived as an "autistic trait" or an obsessive-compulsive aspect to be extinguished when, in fact, it may well be a very positive strategy to aid your child in social interactions.

It should be acknowledged that your child's employ of movie talk is an independently discovered coping mechanism created by someone who, to some degree, recognizes his own limitations and is seeking to ingratiate with "the norm." In someone for whom socialization comes with unpredictable twists and turns, that's a noble endeavor indeed.

In concert with your child, spend time viewing the media segments from which he draws his inspiration. Create drawings, computer images, or written scenarios reflecting the ways in which your child could use the same dialogue (or has already used) in everyday conversation. Try revising or modifying the dialogue slightly if there's a chance of it being clearly recognized by others. Next, partner with your child to compose two columns on a piece of paper—all the known movie talk dialogue your child presently uses in the left-hand column, and in the right-hand column a more commonly used or more acceptable phrase that communicates the same thing. This will require practice, refinement, and reminders, but it's one positive way to build from a strength your child already possesses.

My daughter with autism kissed a boy older than she is because he said he'd give her money—how do I get her to understand the concept of ulterior motives?

This question of understanding ulterior motives is about an unawareness of being taken advantage of, as well as setting one's personal boundaries. The personal boundaries aspect is one that you will need to instill in your child consistently, as you would for any of your children, by setting forth clear expectations in ways your child will best understand. (This includes not accepting money from anyone for anything that hasn't met with your prior approval, especially if it involves bodily contact.)

Remember, there are conditions for social interactions that you may think are common sense, but require teaching and interpreting for the person with autism. Ulterior motives can be challenging for any number of us, particularly if the perpetrator is especially cunning and manipulative. In this example, the boy was relatively unsophisticated and direct: a kiss in exchange for money. In other instances, the situation may be more seductive and not as easily discerned.

You can't anticipate every possible scenario, but, in conjunction with teaching personal boundaries, you can instill within your child the concept of getting a second opinion from a trusted ally if she is uncertain about how best to respond in a situation. Together with your child, draw up a list of potential infractions and threats, and possibly allow your child to illustrate what those situations might look and sound like. Next list all of your child's most trusted allies, the people to whom she can go for a second opinion. You will need to coach your child into realizing that where possible ulterior motives are concerned, there's nothing that requires an immediate reply, nothing that can't wait until a second opinion is sought.

Can adults take advantage of my child because he doesn't question what people tell him and believes they're telling the truth?

Yes—your child with autism is especially vulnerable to manipulative adults for several reasons. First, as the question poses, many individuals on the autism spectrum—children and adults—have difficulty detecting when someone is lying because they are unable to discern eye contact, facial expressions, or body language that might be obvious tip-offs to anyone else. And it's true that many persons with autism accept at face value what someone is saying as the truth because of a tendency to interpret information in ways that are very literal and concrete. Additionally, the child who doesn't speak or isn't fully verbally articulate may be at risk of being a silent victim.

Some very visual ways to teach your child that someone may be lying (and to kick in the second opinion strategy from the preceding inquiry) would be to coach him into looking for two or more of the following happening simultaneously in the other person:

- not making direct eye contact;
- the pupils of the eyes may get narrow from stress;
- crossing and uncrossing arms;
- laughing nervously or laughing more than usual;
- excessive sweating;
- putting one's hands up to the face, or near or covering the mouth;
- subconsciously nodding "yes" when saying "no"; or
- talking too fast.

You can play a fun guessing game with your child to underscore these visual traits, or you can have your child illustrate scenarios in which someone is being deceived. You should also set limits about encounters with strangers in the community with the same cautions as you would for any child.

My child is well liked by his Little League team, but now that he's middle school–aged, I'm starting to see him become more frustrated with his own physical limitations—how do I handle this?

When we are very young, we tend to be more oblivious to the wants and needs of others; we're focused on getting our own needs met, staying out of trouble, and following the rules to the best of our ability. As the child with autism begins to age toward adolescence, his own limitations—which were previously of little consequence—may become glaringly apparent. This may come about due to his own cognizant perceptions, or because his peers have become more sophisticated and critical of others.

In this example, it is the child who has become aware of his difficulty not being as agile or coordinated as he wishes to be (unless he's being overly harsh on himself). Fortunately this child is "well liked," but that may only extend so far in a competitive situation in which scoring points is the goal. In this instance, the child will have to work and train extra hard to achieve a physical prowess on par with his peers; your child will require your help to determine if this kind of investment is sound.

In an alternative scenario, the same child who falls short may need support in discerning how to transform his desire to participate in athletic activities. Does he truly enjoy playing, or would he be willing to serve in an ancillary capacity of some sort, such as assistant coach, manager, timekeeper, or equipment manager? It may be that just participating to some extent would be satisfying; it doesn't necessarily mean actively playing the game. This option may soften the blow for the child who berates himself, finds himself unwanted because of weak skills, or gets cut from the team—all of which could be devastating.

How can I help my child see that the world isn't always fair, and sometimes people do things we don't expect?

No parent wants to see their child fail or be set up for harm of any kind. But, as stated earlier, you cannot possibly anticipate every threatening or upsetting circumstance that might impact your child. And, in thinking about it, would you really want to?

Yes, people lie, deceive, manipulate, and do things that are out of character—some of which is just human nature, and frustratingly so. Are you being fair to your child to perceive her as forever fragile and so susceptible to harm that you seek to micromanage her life and insulate her from what's real? As you're pondering this inevitability, contemplate also the previously discussed concept of the dignity of risk and the minor ways you can allow your child to learn from her own mistakes. There's only so much you can teach as a parent, and sometimes the most enduring life lessons come courtesy of the school of hard knocks. Instead of worrying for the future of your child's interactions, in reflection, you may wish to tally all the ways in which—despite her very sensitive nature—your child is strong and resilient. You may find yourself surprised by the results of this revealing survey with regards to your child's inherent fortitude. Reinforce with your child that you are her ally and will always listen, even as she struggles alongside you to make sense of an oftentimes confusing world.

How do I help my teen with autism who has a couple close friends, but lately doesn't want to spend time with them?

If your teen with autism loses interest in spending time with friends, try to cull from him any information that will help you understand what's happening. Misunderstandings and misinterpretations are common culprits for causing rifts and drifts in relationships—it may have been a situation that was totally avoidable or one with a ready explanation to help smooth things over. Some friends may seem like friends but really aren't *true* friends; does your child know he can trust these friends, and how well do you know them yourself? Finally, if your child's desire to distance himself from his friends persists, you should consider that it might be an indicator (especially in a teenager with autism) of a depressed mood. Don't delay exploring this possibility, and please revisit the chapter on mental health (Chapter 6) for further details.

My teenage son is extremely moral. How do I help him understand when he gets socially isolated because he "tells" on his male peers when they start talking about sex, scantily clad girls, porn, etc.?

Your teen son's moral compass is set high, and there's nothing wrong with his wishing to avoid explicit conversations that make him ill at ease or upset—be happy that he's defined his ethics and values so solidly at such a young age. This is what suits his personal beliefs, but he'll need to be taught the concept of "to each his own" in addition to understanding that—unless harm against someone is intended—he needn't turn in his peers for talking about subjects many male teens tend to find preoccupying. His social isolation may become compounded not just for his autism, but for a developing reputation as a tattletale or "whistle-blower."

One parent in similar circumstances asked, "What can I do or where can I go for an adolescent friend with similar moral coding?" Your son will never be able to escape seeing or hearing material that he finds offensive, but obvious environments in which he might be likely to make connections with others that share his values include:

- religious-related activities and functions,
- YMCA/YWCA activities,
- peer mentoring or Big Brother/Big Sister,
- faith-based discussion groups or book clubs,
- 4-H or other youth-oriented organizations.
- Boy Scouts/Girl Scouts. and
- various charity-based or volunteer-affiliated organizations.

My teen with autism has never had a romantic attachment, and says she doesn't care to. Should I believe her, and is this a problem?

If your teen with autism says she has never—yet—had a romantic attachment, your first inclination should be to accept what she's telling you as the truth. She may be unable to relate to members of the opposite sex who are her own age or may not find them as sensitive or stimulating as she would wish. That doesn't mean never say never, but the more you coax, cajole, and press her about it, the more likely she is to resist the notion like most teens would. The second part of her statement, that she doesn't care to have a relationship, may only be to reinforce her disinterest at present. As to whether it's a problem depends on what you're willing to accept—whose problem would it be if she decides to continue as she is? Autistic or not, some people are comfortable in relationships with others, some people are perfectly happy being in their own company, and still others choose both at different times in their lives—and that's okay. Allow your child the luxury of deciding for herself which she'd prefer to be.

My child has a romantic crush on a girl that is not welcomed, and he has been discouraged by her. How do I help him understand this rejection when he insists she likes him?

Unrequited love can be a painful experience for anyone; for the young person with autism, it can be confusing, awkward, and devastating. This may be compounded by the inability to interpret social cues such as body language, facial expressions, sarcasm, and the meaning of unreturned phone calls and emails. To support your child through this difficult passage, sit with him to develop a list of the indicators by which he believes someone would demonstrate mutual affection. Though you may be surprised by his naiveté, you may suggest that you add to it based on your experiences. If this is too personal, allow a less intimidating approach by discussing (or viewing) fictional characters that were mutually affectionate and what made them so. Next, develop a list of the ways someone might communicate their disinterest or discouragement, and discuss how some or all aspects of that list may have personal application for your child's circumstances.

Your child with autism may be so enthralled with the seduction of wanting to be wanted and loved that he may violently refuse your reasonable rationales. You will need to enforce these concepts, especially if the other party has been clear about not wanting to be bothered any longer. It may be that your child hasn't yet received the relationship-terminating signs that his fictional point of reference received, and so he still thinks the coast is clear to continue pursuing it. The danger is that, sometimes, persons on the autism spectrum have become so blindly infatuated that they take drastic measures like stalking and threatening to harm the other party or attempting suicide. You'll want to be hypervigilant to any such signs in your child, and communicate in no uncertain terms the potential ramifications of those actions if he broaches them. Whereas a typical teen might vent by making an emotional statement that they have no intention of enacting, the teen with autism is most likely to say what he means, and mean what he says.

Chapter 11

SCHOOL SUCCESS

- Does my child with autism need to attend a special school?
- Is any one type of teaching more beneficial than another for my child?
- How do I prepare my child for the first day of school?
- What can I do to help my child's teachers understand his autism better?
- Should I make a presentation to my child's class, or the entire school, about her autism?
- How do I deal with my concerns about the school environment overwhelming my child during the day?
- How come they're calling it *inclusion* when my child is seated away from the other kids?
- My child's teacher has a visual schedule for the class, but my child still has anxiety about certain aspects of it—what do I do?
- Why does my child tell his teacher that he understands something when he shows (through his work) that he clearly doesn't?
- How do I handle it when my child is being picked on by other kids?
- What do I do if I feel my child is being bullied by a teacher?
- Why is my child's teacher constantly sending him to "time out" or the principal's office every day? Now he acts out deliberately so he can get out of class this way!
- What do I do if my child thinks his teacher doesn't like him because his teacher doesn't call on him?
- How do I explain to my child's teacher that my child bit her because she was expecting to receive her report card on a specific day (the day of the incident) and never did?
- What do I do if my child is telling me he is being essentially locked in a closet during the school day for "being bad"?
- How do I handle it if my child has lots of issues with homework?
- Why does my child come home from school nearly every day and go ballistic, flapping his hands and screeching or trashing his bedroom? His teacher says he is basically fine during the day—is this my fault?
- What is IDEA?
- What is an IEP?
- Do I have to wait for the school to schedule the IEP meeting?
- Is there anything that is a "must have" for my child's IEP that is sometimes forgotten?

■ How do I keep the focus on my child when he is expected to have traditional IEP goals?

■ If I'm not happy with my child's IEP do I still have to sign it?

■ Other than transferring my child to another school, do I have any other options if I feel like my school district's not "getting it"?

■ When should a parent choose to homeschool?

■ Knowing that school is the "best" place for socialization, should a parent ever consider homeschooling for a child who lacks social skills and needs to be around other kids?

■ What do I do if I'm concerned about my child losing skills he acquired in school over summer vacation?

Does my child with autism need to attend a special school?

First and foremost, kids are kids; and all children with autism are entitled to be fully included in typical classrooms with their peers to the greatest extent possible. Inclusion benefits both kinds of kids: the child with autism has natural opportunities to learn about educational and social expectations as modeled by classmates, and the classmates can learn about compassionate accommodations and sensitivity for diversity from the child with autism. However, strategies and adaptations will need to be in place to support the child with autism and help her blend as seamlessly as possible.

Depending on your child's strengths, needs, and abilities, she may require additional educational support in the form of a teacher's aide, tutor, therapist, or intensive instruction for some curriculum areas in an alternative classroom setting, within the school, for portions of her day. "Special schools" for children with autism exist only because regular schools haven't yet mastered the autism essentials, many of which are set forth in this book.

Is any one type of teaching more beneficial than another for my child?

The "type" of teaching that will most benefit your child with autism will emanate from the educator who is:

- willing to learn,
- loves kids,
- respects your child's sensitivities,
- gladly implements compassionate accommodations,
- offers creative solutions,
- collaborates with you and your child,
- will advocate for your child's needs,

- wants your child to succeed, and
- expects the best from each child and treats them all equally.

These qualities, coupled with educational and treatment strategies tailored to meet your child's needs, will poise your child for a happy school experience.

How do I prepare my child for the first day of school?

You should prepare your child for the first day of a new school year beginning on the last day of school before summer vacation. This should include an introduction to the new classroom teacher (if there is a new teacher), a tour of the new classroom, how to get there from the school entrance, how to find the bathroom, gym, and cafeteria from the new location, and an anticipated classroom schedule and curriculum. Allow your child to spend as much time as possible getting acclimated and absorbing this information.

Taking a video or photographs to document the proceedings will lessen anxiety as the new school year draws near. A personal note from the new teacher with his or her photograph attached is a gracious courtesy that may be reviewed—together with the video or other photos—at any time prior to the start of the new school year. This kind of foreknowledge should bolster your child's comfort level immeasurably. Sharing this information with prospective classmates creates a social opportunity with your child as the point of contact.

What can I do to help my child's teachers understand his autism better?

Knowledge is power, and you should prepare your child's teachers as you did your child (see previous response). One mom offers a solution with which she has had great success:

I type up a personal biography about my daughter and her specific issues and needs. I title it *All About (her name)*. I include a cover sheet with her picture. The biography discusses the following topics: my daughter's diagnoses, likes and dislikes, things she cannot tolerate (sensory stuff), how she learns best, and things that she needs help with (strengths and weaknesses). I also ended it with a thank you and an inspirational quote. I keep it to the point and as direct as possible. I put it in a folder so the teacher can keep it and refer back to it throughout the year. I also make copies of interesting articles that pertain to my child's diagnosis and slip them into the folder. I send new articles and suggestions throughout the year. My daughter's teacher has enjoyed this very much, and it helps clarify what specific needs my child has without going into all of the diagnostic criteria and repeating myself throughout the year. I also give this biography to baby-sitters, therapists, new doctors, and family members.

Should I make a presentation to my child's class, or the entire school, about her autism?

Before you consider this any further, listen to one parent who encountered an impasse in poor judgment with her child's school district concerning confidentiality and rights to disclosure for several students with autism: "The principal of our elementary school 'outed' them in front of two hundred parents at our back-to-school night. Needless to say we had not told our children of their autism diagnosis."

Recall that personal disclosure is a very intimate and personal decision, one that your child should be afforded the opportunity to determine with appropriate consent. Many parents find value in discussing their child's autism with classmates, but what purpose is served by singling out your child's diagnosis in front of her entire class or at a school assembly no matter how gentle or well intentioned it may be? Even if it is done anonymously, most typical kids won't be interested, won't remember, or won't know who is being discussed.

Are there other ways you can promote sensitivity of your child's different way of being that are more subtle? Your child's classmates follow the tone set by their educators and school administration. How is inclusion and respect for diversity promoted in your child's school? Are there opportunities to have discussions with classmates about how we are all more alike than different; and when we are different, what that might look like? You can even use the sensory sensitivity exercises referenced in this book and have dialogues about thinking and learning differently. Can you compromise your desire to incorporate an enhanced sensitivity for your child's needs in school with a quieter approach?

How do I deal with my concerns about the school environment overwhelming my child during the day?

Understand that, every school day, your very sensitive child with autism is struggling to assimilate his environment, attend to the curriculum, and engage socially. It requires hard work and extraordinary effort. This isn't a matter of education—we're talking about survival! Your child should be privately praised for his accomplishments in holding it together under oftentimes very stressful circumstances. In consideration of how your child thinks and learns and processes sensory information differently, brainstorm with him and his educational team about additional coping strategies that will allow him to pace himself throughout the day, maintain some measure of control, and ensure that, wherever possible, he has information about what's coming next.

For example, many kids with autism become totally unhinged by the unpredictable assault of the fire drill alarm; so much so that they can cry, become aggressive, or go numb with anxiety. In what ways can your child gain some control over the situation in terms of the school administration making compassionate accommodations? In many instances, the child is given foreknowledge of the time of the drill in order to play favored music on a Walkman (don't worry, he'll still hear the alarm) or to assume an appointed responsibility such as holding open the classroom door or keeping a head count. In other examples, the alarm in the room (or just outside the room in the hallway) has been muffled to decrease its volume though the alarm still clearly sounds throughout the rest of the building. Perhaps your child and his educational team can develop further compromises. Once determined, ensure that any such measures are detailed and recorded in your child's education plan. In this way, everyone is accountable for being knowledgeable and consistent about how best to support your child's potential to become overwhelmed by his school environment.

How come they're calling it *inclusion* when my child is seated away from the other kids?

Before jumping to conclusions, consult with your child's teacher about why your child is positioned in the room as she is. Your child's teacher may have good reasons for seating your child in a way that may be advantageous to her ability to learn. However, if you, as the parent, have been unaware of your child's seating arrangement and its rationale, then there's been a breakdown in communication somewhere along the way—you should have been apprised of your child's classroom difficulties. Is her seat closer to the teacher, out from under strong lights, or placed free from visual distractions? These are among the questions to pursue as you investigate what's transpired. If you disagree with the circumstances, you may request that a meeting be held to discuss the situation and propose alternatives that may better suit your child's needs.

In some instances, however, teachers may separate children with differences from other children for punitive measures or to prevent any acts of aggression from occurring. In one example, a child on the autism spectrum was seated with his classroom aide at the back of the room at great distance from the other "typical" children—and this child had a visual impairment! Because of the teacher's resistance against including a child with autism in his classroom, the student was not involved, not called on, and could not clearly see any of the visuals used by the teacher such as maps, charts, and illustrations. Yet, because the child was physically in the same room, the school qualified it as "inclusion," and the teacher's tenure precluded him from being reprimanded by a weak administration.

None of the preceding examples are valid reasons for excluding a child from participating in an inclusion classroom setting. Such situations require sensitive discussion to achieve a resolution. Such discussions may involve an outside advocate, counselor, or consultant who specializes in mediating differences of opinion or interpretation of your child's educational requirements.

My child's teacher has a visual schedule for the class, but my child still has anxiety about certain aspects of it—what do I do?

Sequential picture or written schedules are fundamental for assuring all children—and particularly the child with autism—about what to expect, what is expected, and what's coming next. The educator who devises a visual schedule for the entire class is on the right track, it's just that the concept requires tweaking to become individualized to the needs of your child in order to contain and quell her anxiety. If the schedule is too far from your child's seat, or if she needs to get out of her seat to look at it (or is too afraid to ask to get out of her seat to look at it), then its value is not being successfully maximized by your child, and a terrific concept becomes useless to her. In what ways can the classroom teacher's good thinking be improved?

Some ideas might include discarding the posted schedule in favor of issuing personal copies of the schedule to all students, or making certain that your child has a personal copy of the schedule that she may annotate to suit her needs. Your child's anxiety may be stemming from her teacher being too flexible and not following the schedule as posted, or your child may feel lost, anxious, and vulnerable during times when she is out of her main classroom participating in extracurricular classes, lunch, or recess and is without the schedule.

Additionally, are events or adjustments to the schedule noted as far in advance as possible? Does the schedule provide information for just the day, a week at a time, or the whole month? Depending on your child's needs and anxieties, crucial information might be absent from the classroom schedule; maybe her teacher has made reference to a future event that does not appear on the schedule. It may be that, in addition to the classroom schedule, your child would benefit from referring to her own personal schedule for the year that includes indications of birthdays, fire drills, assemblies, report card days, vacations, and early dismissals. Partner with your child and her educators to determine what might best suit her needs with regard to a schedule that promotes her comfort and control.

Why does my child tell his teacher that he understands something when he shows (through his work) that he clearly doesn't?

Your child may be saying one thing but reflecting another through the quality of his schoolwork for a couple reasons. First, what is his relationship like with his classroom teacher? Is it a relationship built on mutual respect, or is it one of intimidation? If no comfort level is apparent, or if the teacher has previously singled out your child by humiliating him in front of others, he may be telling her what she wants to hear to keep her at arm's length and have as little contact as possible.

On the other hand—and especially if your child likes his teacher—he may be telling her what she wants to hear because many kids on the autism spectrum are "pleasers." That is, they wish to avoid conflict at all costs in order to keep the adults in their lives happy. This may mean your child is consenting to something he doesn't clearly understand, or agreeing to something he hasn't yet had the time to fully process because he's feeling an imposed pressure to content his teacher in the moment. (You may also see the child with a weakened self-image portray himself in this manner as well.)

You can help the situation by privately counseling your child about this concept in ways that he will best understand. The teacher may also wish to communicate to your child in writing, instead of verbally in the moment, and request that your child respond in writing (or typing) by the end of the day or before a natural transition to gain a more accurate impression of his learning experience.

How do I handle it when my child is being picked on by other kids?

There are no circumstances under which you should allow your child to be bullied—and you should disbelieve others who tell you that all kids go through it, that it will "toughen up" your child, or that it will shame your child into compliance. As one who is possessed with a different way of being that predisposes him to be inherently gentle and exquisitely sensitive, your child is already vulnerable as an easy mark and a target for abuse, especially beginning with the middle school years when he is more likely to be perceived as an outsider.

By today's standards, most school districts have a no-tolerance bullying policy. Be certain you have a copy of the policy and are well aware of its protocols. Discuss with your child, in ways that he will best understand, what bullying might look like (including verbal and physical harassment) and ensure that he knows full well how to respond to such situations. This kind of prevention—not intervention—is crucial, but may also raise your child's anxiety level about being in the school environment; you'll need to reread and review the protocols with your child to provide comfort and assurances.

Just because your child's school district has a no-bullying policy in place doesn't mean bullying doesn't occur or that it gets reported when it does. You'll need to be vigilant in insisting that your child's school staff be observant and willing to intercede should they detect any wrongdoing. Your child himself may not be telling what's occurring to him either because he is too traumatized and upset, because he thinks it's his fault, or because he believes the threats made against him if he tells. If you suspect this may be the case, you'll need to lovingly support your child to get him to confide in you; examine his body at bath time for marks, scratches, and bruises; and provide consistent assurances for his safety and well-being. Finally, ensure that no-bullying measures are written into your child's education plan for reasons of accountability and consistency (more on this plan, or IEP, shortly).

What do I do if I feel my child is being bullied by a teacher?

Kids with autism are not universally embraced in every teacher's classroom, and there are some educators who resent or hold in contempt children they may view as having behavioral problems or requiring extra time and effort. As unbelievable as it may sound, there are cases of children with autism being teased and abused by the very adults who should be protecting them from such flagrancies. Not only is this breach of trust inexcusable, it can cause your child extreme emotional distress that may manifest in symptoms of depression and post-traumatic stress disorder.

Being bullied by a teacher may go unreported by your child because he thinks all adults are right, perfect, and not to be challenged, especially teachers. Your child may not even interpret what's happening as bullying; he just knows he dislikes a certain teacher, doesn't learn well in that person's presence, or even becomes sick at the mere mention of that teacher's name. Even the educator who is well intended and trying to motivate your child may, in fact, be wrongly and unduly pressuring your child, or humiliating him with what the teacher may see only as coaxing or inspiring encouragement.

If you suspect that your child is being bullied by one of his educators, contact that person immediately to discuss the situation. Make crystal clear your position regarding what you will and will not tolerate, and substantiate your claims with reports of changes in your child's behavior. If you clash or are left feeling dissatisfied, contact your child's school principal for a private meeting to discuss the matter. Do not accept any excuse or convenient rationale for inappropriate and insensitive conduct by an educator in whom your child's care is entrusted.

Why is my child's teacher constantly sending him to "time out" or the principal's office every day? Now he acts out deliberately so he can get out of class this way!

Your child's teacher is constantly sending him to the principal's office because she is in need of support, training, and resources she either hasn't received or needs assistance in applying to a classroom setting. Sending your child to the principal's office is a quick and easy resolution that provides your child's teacher with a hands-off approach that relieves her of responsibility but, ultimately, is a disservice to your child, as you've observed. It also sets a negative precedent: no student gets sent to the principal's office for good behavior! Your child probably doesn't mind the interruption because he senses that he is disliked by his teacher regardless, so for him it's as much a respite as it is for his teacher.

Arrange a time to sit down with your child's teacher and anyone else you think would be beneficial such as the principal, director of special education, and the school psychologist, to discuss the issues and how you might emphasize *prevention* (keeping your child in class, interested and attentive) instead of *intervention* (having him languish in the principal's office, excluded from receiving the education to which he is entitled). It may be tempting to enter into such a discussion with an accusatory tone, but if you can be empathetic to the teacher's position of feeling ill supported, be prepared to offer easily implemented solutions and direct assistance to that educator such as autism-specific resources, reading and viewing materials, and training opportunities—it will greatly enhance her comfort level, foster better communications between you both, and the trickle-down effect will improve the manner in which the teacher interacts with your child.

Your child will also require counseling to communicate to him that both you and his teacher expect that he stay in class outside of breaks, and that acting out for the purpose of being excused to the principal's office is no longer an option. Instead, inform your child of the new measures being taken to help everyone feel at ease in the classroom, and reinforce the ways in which your child can better pace himself during the school day in order to better attend and maintain in the classroom environment.

What do I do if my child thinks his teacher doesn't like him because his teacher doesn't call on him?

In the eyes of the young child with autism who desires to please, his teacher is an authority figure on par with the Almighty. If your child has communicated that he doesn't think his teacher likes him, it can be devastating and cause internal issues of inferiority and damaged esteem. First, is your child clearly certain about the rules for raising your hand if you know the answer and waiting to be called on? Many teachers will not call on those children who do not correctly practice this classroom etiquette; it may need to be taught and practiced with your child. Try to ascertain if there's been a communication breakdown here and if this is the root of the problem.

Next, knowing your child as well as you do, is it possible that he's being especially sensitive? Is he being called on as much as anyone else, or is he raising his hand for every question the teacher asks—whether or not he knows the answer? If this is the case, you can see how he could misinterpret his teacher's actions and the desire to give other children a chance.

Finally, talk with your child's teacher and determine how to resolve the issue. (Make sure that she's not refraining from calling on your child because she doesn't like him.) Share your child's perception with his teacher and discuss ways she might alleviate any hard feelings. It may require reviewing the protocol for raising one's hand in class, which doesn't guarantee you'll be selected to respond. A good way to approach this, that doesn't single out your child, is for the teacher to revisit this concept with the entire class in a verbal and visual review.

How do I explain to my child's teacher that my child bit her because she was expecting to receive her report card on a specific day (the day of the incident) and never did?

This is another circumstance in which prevention should prevail before intervention. Most likely, this isn't the first time your child has bitten anyone, let alone an adult. In fairness to your child's teacher, the teacher should have been apprised of the potential for this to occur—and under what conditions—well in advance of the incident, no matter how uncommon it may be for your child to engage in this extreme communication of her frustration. If communication between you and your child's teacher has flowed in a reciprocal way, you both should have also previously discussed how sudden changes in schedule can impact your child's expectations and mood without warning. This will help your child's teacher be conscious of giving advance notice to all classroom students about any impending schedule adjustments.

Your child's teacher is a human being, though. As such, she cannot possibly anticipate every event that may upset and distress your child. Your child requires your counsel, in ways she will best understand, about flexibility within a set schedule, and will need opportunities for breaks and downtime in order to pace herself prior to a blowup. Additionally, under no circumstances is it okay for your child to bite anyone. You'll need to communicate this loud and clear, and impose fair but firm disciplinary measures should it continue. Concurrently, teach your child alternative ways to communicate her upset in order to alleviate future such situations that have great potential to stigmatize her by giving her a reputation as a "biter."

What do I do if my child is telling me he is being essentially locked in a closet during the school day for "being bad"?

If your child is telling you he is being locked in a closet during the day (*locked* being the operative word), remove him from school immediately pending an investigation that you should initiate by contacting the school principal. Next, find a strong parent advocate, hire an attorney, or consult with a solicitor willing to represent you gratis. This is a serious situation, and your child is being managed and contained—not educated—using an aversive technique called *seclusion*.

Not only was he being abused and traumatized, you will need to ascertain if he had access to a toilet, water, and food during the time he was in the closet. You'll also need to determine if this occurred daily and for what duration of time, exactly who put him there, and where such a procedure was documented as acceptable. Additionally, did your child injure himself while in the closet, and was he mistreated in other ways he hasn't reported? If your child's conduct is so extreme that the school feels the need to use this type of punishment, you certainly should have been informed of their challenges to educate him long before learning of it directly from your child.

How do I handle it if my child has lots of issues with homework?

Homework is problematic for a number of children with autism. Some take homework so seriously that they become overwrought with anxiety that renders them incapable of doing their best—even though they ordinarily may know how to respond. They may, instead, tantrum, wail, or hyperventilate like it's a life-or-death situation. Some reasons why kids on the autism spectrum may find homework challenging could include the following:

- disorganization by your child (or you!) that causes her to poorly plan time to complete homework;
- feeling overwhelmed with too much homework;
- not understanding what's expected because it hasn't been communicated in ways in which she thinks, learns, and processes information;
- understanding what's expected but feeling offended or insulted when she must complete work she's already shown that she knows;
- upset over homework that is verbally reviewed in class, which leaves her feeling inferior or stereotyped;
- being in a perfectionism mode that creates frustration and delays, resulting in excessive erasing, tearing up work papers, or melting down; and
- being expected to handwrite everything when handwriting is uncomfortable, illegible, or very difficult.

Ensure that you discuss these or any additional homework issues with your child and her teacher to determine the source of your child's angst. Map out, on a schedule, manageable portions of time in which to realistically complete homework assignments. Work out a compromise with the teacher if your child already demonstrates mastery of the homework concepts. Discuss alternative ways to submit homework if handwriting or perfectionism is an obstacle, such as typing, emailing, or verbally recording the information. Underscore with your child that perfect answers are not expected in all cases. Reinforce with her teacher how your child best thinks and learns—can her passion(s) be used to decode homework that's challenging to understand? Partner with your child and her teacher to brainstorm further by building on these and other strategies.

Why does my child come home from school nearly every day and go ballistic, flapping his hands and screeching or trashing his bedroom? His teacher says he is basically fine during the day—is this my fault?

Let's remember that we are all more alike than different. Many kids on the autism spectrum are working hard to blend and assimilate during the school day. A lot of kids with autism say they just want to be accepted like everyone else. This requires extreme concentration and determination. Reflect on all that can transpire during a typical school day for someone on the autism spectrum. In addition to attempting to learn, your child must deal with:

- social expectations during unstructured time such as recess and lunch,
- environmental stimuli that may be distracting or painful,
- changes in scheduling or routine,
- new or changing educational expectations,
- unchallenging educational expectations,
- changes in classroom dynamics (teacher or student absences), and
- possibly humiliation or embarrassment from being bullied by peers or educators .

Now think about all the ways in which most "neuro-typical" folks pace themselves during a typical workday in order to make things more pleasant and bearable. These might involve bathroom, cigarette, coffee, and snack breaks, going out to lunch, chatting by the water cooler, getting some fresh air or walking, reading, or surfing the Internet. If we denied anyone the preceding coping strategies, and demanded instead a rigid or standardized conformity by which their time was regulated, there'd be a revolt! This would likely manifest in "behaviors" that would be labeled as verbally and physically aggressive, or noncompliant.

The following are some discreet, natural-appearing tactics you can recommend for your child so that he, too, can pace himself to avert a meltdown during the day or so that he can prevent unleashing all of that pent-up frustration on arriving home:

- bathroom breaks;
- water fountain breaks;
- quiet reading breaks;
- listening to calming music on headphones;
- using the computer;
- changing the water bottle for the classroom's gerbil, hamster, or lizard;
- delivering attendance forms or other papers to the office or another room during class when the halls are quiet; and
- coming in a minute or two before everyone else from recess, gym, lunch, or some other crowded, noisy environment that may require sensory de-escalation.

What is IDEA?

IDEA is the acronym for the Individuals with Disabilities Education Act. IDEA is the federal law that guarantees that your child with autism be provided with a free and appropriate education (called *FAPE*). In addition to autism, IDEA also covers kids with mental retardation; hearing, vision, or speech/language impairments; serious emotional issues; orthopedic impairment; traumatic brain injury; other health-related impairment; or a specific learning disability.

IDEA also requires that, wherever possible, all children should be included and educated in the least restrictive environment (LRE), which means alongside their typical peers in regular classrooms. Thus, your child should not be taught in environments that exclude him from his classmates because of his autism. (Not so long ago, kids with differences were isolated in segregated "special ed" environments because they were labeled as intellectually inferior.)

IDEA mandates the national Early Intervention program for children with disabilities who qualify (referenced in Chapter 2). IDEA also provides for your child with autism to receive an evaluation for educational services and supports, for a formal plan to be drawn up to document those supports (the IEP), and for safeguards to be in place that are accessible to parents who disagree with the proceedings (more on this later).

What is an IEP?

Once your child's eligibility under IDEA is determined via an educational evaluation, any accommodations to support her capacity to be productive and learn with her typical peers in an education setting are formally recorded in a document known as the *individualized education plan*, or IEP. Within thirty calendar days of the date your child has been determined eligible, an IEP team should be established that may be composed of you and your spouse, a regular education teacher, a special education teacher, a decision-making school representative (such as the principal), someone who can interpret the evaluation results in terms of your child's education needs, and others with special expertise such as a parent advocate or consultants who specialize in autism or writing IEPs. Your child may also attend the meeting but be forewarned that oftentimes deficit-based topics may be openly and insensitively discussed depending on the team's composition.

The IEP is a blueprint for your child's educators that will individualize your child's strengths and needs, and includes realistically achievable goals, described in steps, by which your child's progress may be measured incrementally. The IEP document will also indicate the start date for services, the duration of services, and any revisions. The IDEA category, "program modifications and specially designed instruction," for example, should itemize the learning and environmental accommodations your child requires and should be listed as such in the IEP. There must also be a statement indicating why your child's educational placement represents the least restrictive environment.

The final document should include a cover sheet and a sign-in attendance page, a statement of your child's eligibility, a space for you to sign acknowledging that you have been informed of your rights (called *procedural safeguards*), your contact information, any special considerations that may hinder your child's ability to learn, and summaries of your child's strengths and needs. You may request a blank copy of the IEP form in advance of the meeting; and an Internet search of the words "sample IEP" will lead you to any number of websites that will give you helpful hints and strategies, provide ideas for crafting goals, and show you what well-composed IEPs for kids with differences should look like.

Do I have to wait for the school to schedule the IEP meeting?

The completed IEP must be implemented within ten school days, and must also be formally reviewed at least annually. If you have not heard from your child's school within this time frame, call the person who conducted the original evaluation or ask to speak with the school principal to schedule the meeting. It is advisable that you document the date and time of your phone contacts and what was discussed, and follow up with a letter reiterating the information as you understand it. Your child's completed and mutually agreed-upon IEP must be in place prior to the start of each new school year so that his educators have a map to guide them in consistently providing your child with goals, accommodations, and opportunities for educational success.

Is there anything that's a "must have" for my child's IEP that is sometimes forgotten?

If your child's way of communicating is too often interpreted as stereotypical autism "behaviors" that interfere with his ability to learn (or precludes his classmates from learning), it is tempting for many educators to rely on old-school methods of punishment and intimidation to force your child to comply and behave. Remember that compliance for the sake of compliance does not equal success; not understanding the reasoning for your child's communications presupposes that he is a bad kid and a behavior problem. This mind-set perpetuates a lack of presumed intellect and initiates a self-fulfilling prophecy that may solidify your child's negative reputation early on.

If this is the case, it is very important for you and any allies you may have requested to participate in the IEP meeting (including a parent advocate who has "been there, done that") to persist in imploring the IEP team to keep the focus on your child and his strengths and needs. Because you know your child best, you can decode your child's behaviors in terms of expressions of communication. Do not hesitate to do so by discussing:

- the presumption of intellect (including not talking about your child in front of him),
- sensory sensitivities,
- ways in which your child interprets information literally or visually,
- physical limitations,
- emotional upsets, and
- self-soothing techniques.

Exploring these aspects of your child's autism will help dissuade the IEP team from fostering preconceived misperceptions about your parenting skills or your child's capabilities derived from myths and stereotypes. Ensure that any behavioral support plan is stated in positive terms without punitive consequences for your child unless fair discipline is called for, per Chapter 9. Remember that your child's attempts to express himself have tremendous potential to be taken out of context or completely misinterpreted; your child is depending on you to represent him as a human being and not a behavior problem.

How do I keep the focus on my child when he is expected to have traditional IEP goals?

Here is the perfect opportunity to employ the three essential tenets of this book: presume intellect, practice prevention instead of intervention, and foster self-advocacy. As stated in the previous question's answer, ensure that any and all preventive measures are discussed *and* documented so that there's accountability for accommodating your child's needs. Here's an example of a measurable IEP goal written in a traditional style: "Jared will give direct eye contact one-on-one in conversation 80 percent of the time." First, does Jared even understand the rationale for making eye contact—has that concept been taught? Will it be taught through written narrative, role-playing, watching videos, or some other method? Is there a way to build in a natural incentive by including his most passionate of interests? Next, is making eye contact something he can do comfortably and still listen and respond without being overwhelmed or distracted? What is his relationship with the person(s) requesting his eye contact—is there motivation to look at her or him? And has that person assessed themselves and the environment for sensory sensitivity triggers such as bad breath, too much cologne, or irritating background noise?

Rewriting the goal from a respectful, relationship-based approach, it might better read: "Given the implementation of the documented preventive measures, Jared will learn the social protocol for making eye contact, and choose to either give direct eye contact or give directional attendance (a fancy way of saying he'll approximate eye contact or look in the direction of his communication partner) 80 percent of the time." This re-envisioning of IEP goals:

- emphasizes prevention over intervention,
- gives your child personal choice,
- fosters self-advocacy through self-knowledge and self-awareness,
- reduces everyone's frustrations (your child's included),
- eventually reduces the need for intensive services,
- allows the team to focus on other priorities,
- deters everyone from negatively perceiving your child as "noncompliant," and
- creates an opportunity for success.

A similar perspective can be used when writing any number of IEP goals that will compel your child's education team to think sensitively in terms of prevention and respect.

If I'm not happy with my child's IEP do I still have to sign it?

There will always be kinks to iron out during the IEP process; however, the IDEA provides parents with procedural safeguards in the event your child's individualized education plan comes into dispute. You do not have to sign your child's IEP if you disagree with it in whole or even in part. Do not feel obligated or pressured to endorse the document with your signature even if you qualify it with notations—this is not required either. Instead, request that the IEP meeting be continued or rescheduled until any disagreements can be resolved amicably. In fact, you may request that an IEP meeting be convened at any time during your child's school career—even outside of the mandated IEP anniversary date.

If you are in conflict with your child's school district but wish to avoid formal action at present, a savvy parent advocate may be a great resource and ally to you in navigating difficult circumstances. The National Parent to Parent Network, referenced in Chapter 2, may be a source for finding a local parent advocate, as may be your closest Autism Society of America chapter (start by looking at their national website at www.autism-society.org).

Other than transferring my child to another school, do I have any other options if I feel like my school district's not "getting it"?

When your child's education is in dispute, your legal recourse, provided by IDEA, may include a formal impartial due process hearing, presided over by a hearing officer. You can request such a hearing in writing. (Hearing officers are employed by your state government's education office of dispute resolution, and may be of varied backgrounds such as former attorneys, education administrators, or psychologists.)

Once your request for an impartial due process hearing has been received by your child's school district, the district has five days to forward your request to the office of dispute resolution, and the hearing is to be scheduled within thirty days of your request. Unless she is a danger to herself and others, during this time your child is to remain in her current educational placement without disruption. At the hearing, both parties will present their side of the situation to the hearing officer, similar to court proceedings. The hearing officer has forty-five days after your request for a hearing within which to render his or her decision. This decision may be appealed by either side and taken to an appeals panel within thirty days, which must render a decision within thirty days of the appeal review request. If the dispute persists, IDEA provides you with the right to file a federal case in any U.S. district court.

The premier website for keeping informed and up to date on your child's educational rights is hosted by special education lawyer, Peter Wright, Esq., at www.wrightslaw.org

When should a parent choose to homeschool?

There is no blanket response to the question of homeschooling—the decision to homeschool is one that is personal and individualized to the needs of each family and the social, emotional, and educational needs of each child with autism. Parents who have elected to home-school may do so for these reasons:

- They feel more knowledgeable about their child's autism than the school district.
- They feel better able to meet their child's needs in a more intimate environment.
- They have decided to temporarily educate their child for safety or other reasons prior to reintroducing him back to his school district.
- They desire greater input and control over their child's educational curriculum.
- They don't have the time, energy, or interest to battle the system.
- Their child is being persistently bullied and there is not sufficient support or resolution by the school district for the child.
- They have access to the kinds of resources and materials not provided for by the school district.
- Their child has indicated the desire to be removed from the school district.
- They have had success in educating their other children in homeschooling.

- They can create innovative opportunities to build on their child's passions.

Homeschooling can be a challenging but rewarding experience for parents who decide to undertake it, and many children with a variety of different ways of being thrive when they feel safe and comfortable in an alternative environment. Begin by learning about the options through a state or local homeschooling organization, or by doing an Internet search for websites such as the National Home Education Network. One caveat, though, is that every time a parent removes a child with special needs from school, the district is being sent the message that they are "off the hook" and absolved of the responsibility to improve and better learn how to serve kids who require a range of adaptations and accommodations. However, there are those instances in which parents feel they simply have no other alternative.

Knowing that school is the "best" place for socialization, should a parent ever consider homeschooling for a child who lacks social skills and needs to be around other kids?

The answer to this question depends on who is determining that school is the best place for socialization. It's true that, as your child grows and matures, school becomes as much about social opportunities as it is about learning. But if homeschooling is considered the alternative, in what context is the child with autism able to flourish socially if he feels inept or awkward or is shunned and singled out?

As you have read in the chapters about making social connections and valuing passions, there are myriad opportunities for your child to engage with others and to experience success in doing so—success that need not necessarily occur in a school environment. Your child's school years have the potential to greatly impact his self-esteem and ability to transition to adulthood with a sense of purpose; to contribute and join with the big, overwhelming, unyielding world. When reflecting on their childhood and adolescence, many adults on the autism spectrum relate feelings of inadequacy, harassment, and worthlessness leading to the mental health issues discussed in Chapter 6.

If your child's social experiences at school are not only preventing him from learning but are causing him to harbor harmful or destructive thoughts, homeschooling may be the best course of action if no other remedy is viable. Autistic or not, we all require communion in the form of human contact but that does not mean, as the question implies, that your child needs to be around other kids who are not compassionate and accepting of his way of being. Socialization opportunities for homeschoolers can include church, organized clubs, classes of all kinds, Boy or Girl Scouts, and other formal and informal activities. On the other hand, if your child has at least one ally in school that "gets" him unconditionally, that relationship can make all the difference in the world.

What do I do if I'm concerned about my child losing skills he acquired in school over summer vacation?

Summer vacation presents challenges for many kids with autism because of the loss of predictable schedules and academic routine in favor of broad blocks of unstructured time in which things can get out of hand, as they might for any idle kid. Your child with autism will benefit greatly from your ability to provide a predictable routine like that he experienced at school through a day care program, summer camp, or possibly an extended school year program.

Many camps are geared toward specific areas of personal passion or talent that might be attractive to your child if he or she is athletic, musical, or artistic. Other camps cater specifically to serving children with different ways of being or special needs by reinforcing certain skills including social, educational and avocational. Parents that you might connect with through your child's school, local autism group, or parent support groups can give you leads about summer recreational programming or campsites in your area, what kinds of activities are offered, and staff training and qualifications. The Internet is also a resource by which you may further investigate the reputation of any such campground.

An extended school year (ESY) program might be available through your school district if you fear your child is regressing in his ability to retain and demonstrate what he has learned academically or socially as it relates to goals identified in his IEP. Such regression in abilities should also be monitored by your child's educators at periodic intervals throughout the school year. The ESY program can look drastically different between school districts, and some schools may be more willing to accommodate than others (in best case scenarios, a school might even fund a summer camp program for your child that would focus on educational and social skills). It is advisable that you not wait until May or June to understand your school district's policy about ESY but, as a precaution, make it part of your child's IEP team discussions from the start.

Chapter 12

YOUNG ADULTHOOD AND BEYOND

- What would the average person with autism say is the best thing about being on the autism spectrum?
- What would the average person with autism say is the hardest thing about being on the autism spectrum?
- Is it okay to want to keep my child living at home forever—will this hurt him socially?
- Will my child be able to live independently someday?
- My child is nineteen and still needs help bathing and getting dressed—will this always be the case?
- Will my child be able to drive a car at age sixteen?
- Because my child thinks and behaves differently, how do I keep him from being misperceived by law enforcement?
- What do I do if he does get in trouble with the law?
- How do I help my child understand the sexual feelings he is having?
- My son is getting more and more interested in girls—how do I teach him to use self-control and to be respectful of others' boundaries?
- Can someone be autistic and gay? My teenage son doesn't seem interested in females, but will comment on attractive male TV stars?
- Will my daughter with autism be able to conceive children as an adult woman, especially given the medications she takes?
- With the struggles my child is having in elementary school, is there any hope for him in junior high, high school, and, one day, college?
- How do I help my child plan for college?
- What particular colleges are best at serving my child's needs?
- How do I deal with feeling scared that my child will be exposed to drugs on campus?
- Will my child be able to have a job?
- What can I do to help my child prepare for a job interview?
- Is my child obligated to disclose her autism to prospective employers?
- What can I do for my child who is despondent about always being passed over by employers?
- I know my child is smart, so why is he only being hired as a janitor at a fast-food restaurant?
- My child has autism and a mental health diagnosis—how can I help her deal with both in adulthood?
- Will my child grow out of autism by adulthood?
- I have heard several news stories about parents murdering their kids with autism—why is this happening?
- What is *person-centered planning* and how can it benefit my child?
- Can I appoint someone to be my child's legal guardian?
- What will become of my child after I die?

What would the average person with autism say is the best thing about being on the autism spectrum?

Adults on the autism spectrum can have unique perspectives of the world, creatively interpreted through their enhanced sensory sensitivities; this can manifest in having an eye for all the little details that go ignored or unseen by others. Many are ingenious problem solvers because they are able to perceive circumstances in ways that are clever and uncommon. Those who think in pictures and movies may even be able to preconceive or visualize something prior to its execution in three dimensions. As discussed in the chapter about valuing passions, when someone with autism is interested in something, he or she becomes an expert on the subject with oftentimes encyclopedic knowledge. Others are good with words, languages, poetry, music, and numbers. Of those asked this question, most self-advocates might say they relish their nontraditional, nonjudgmental way of being in the world replete with its frustrating confusion and moments of startling clarity.

What would the average person with autism say is the hardest thing about being on the autism spectrum?

Several things, not just one, would likely be ranked as hardest about being autistic: (1) the belief that autism equals intellectual inferiority or mental retardation, (2) the persistence of antiquated myths and stereotypes about being without empathy or social connectedness, (3) the insensitivity and lack of acceptance from those with intolerance for diversity, (4) the influx of people who presume to speak on behalf of those with autism but are not autistic themselves, and (5) the message that if you have autism you are broken and need to be fixed or cured—much like trying to change someone who is naturally left-handed into a right-handed person—until there are no more people like you left in the world. To quote one self-advocate who echoes the sentiments of so many others, "Autism is not something which conceals my 'true nature' behind some impenetrable barrier; rather, it permeates my nature and is an inseparable part of who I am."

Is it okay to want to keep my child living at home forever—will this hurt him socially?

If we look at this question in a different light, we see that what you really want is to protect him from experiencing any hurt at the hands of an unyielding and unforgiving world. As a parent, your concern feels justifiable, motivated by a fear of the unknown, because you love your child, know him best, and understand how to get his needs met. (Indeed, these very sentiments were dismissed in the days when specialists argued that all children with developmental differences should be institutionalized.)

If your child was typical, would you want to insulate him from the world by allowing him to live at home forever? Of course not, and he would want his own space the same as anyone else. Your child needs a social circle beyond his relationship with you in order to learn and grow as a person, even if it means having just one ally in his life that understands unconditionally and will help him navigate life. Remember that you should foster self-advocacy and that requires exercising the previously discussed dignity of risk in endeavoring independence.

Will my child be able to live independently someday?

The adult child with autism has the right to live as independently as possible, although there are many challenges to making that happen. Begin planning while your child is young by:
  • connecting with other parents;
  • talking to adults with autism;

- contacting local, statewide, and national autism groups (some of which are listed at the back of this book);
- writing/meeting your legislators to express the need to fund individualized housing for your child and others;
- navigating the ins and outs of your housing authority protocols;
- investigating funding streams, formal and informal, that could be tapped; and
- reading about how other adults with autism and their families are making it happen.

It may be that your child will require assistance, support, roommates, or a romantic partnership in order to dwell on her own away from your home.

My child is nineteen and still needs help bathing and getting dressed—will this always be the case?

If your child has a physical disability that precludes her from bathing and dressing independently, she may, indeed, always require some measure of physical assistance unless there is some technology that might enhance her independence. If this is not the case, is her need for required assistance a lack of understanding that needs to be taught in ways she will best understand, or is her need for required assistance a learned helplessness because no one has fully presumed her intellect? This is what you must first determine prior to knowing how best to proceed. If you have subscribed to the stereotypes about the intellectual inferiority of people with autism, it could very well be that this perceived helplessness is your child's way of reflecting back what others have projected on her—it's called exercising control, and it's a communication that implores, "see me as the competent person I am."

If none of these instances apply, you may want to contact your county's local Human Services agency for suggestions, strategies and recommendations from therapists, home care assistants, and respite providers. It may also be that nurses and other professionals who provide care to persons with disabilities or the elderly have sound ideas to support improving your child's self-care routines.

Will my child be able to drive a car at age sixteen?

While your child with autism may desire to enhance his independence by learning to drive, the reality may be that he is lacking the physical eye–hand–foot coordination, rapid-response reflexes, and split-second, decision-making thought processes that operating a motor vehicle can require at any given moment. Compounding this is that, even if your child knows the rules of the road explicitly, it doesn't mean everyone else abides by those rules as diligently (or legally), which can lead to confusion, road rage, disorientation, and accidents.

None of this, of course, is your child's fault, though the feeling of failure and not keeping par with his peers may sting nonetheless. If you are able to work closely with your child at every free opportunity to practice driving in a safe area, do so. If you honestly believe your child and driving are not a good match, shift your focus to attaining a similar sense of independence by learning completely and thoroughly how to access public transportation such as buses and subways, taxi cabs, and other types of low- or no-cost transportation options in your community.

Because my child thinks and behaves differently, how do I keep him from being misperceived by law enforcement?

If you know your child to be aggressive, impulsive, or someone who elopes (runs away) regularly, it may behoove you and your family to make contact with your local law enforcement officers now. While improvements are occurring slowly in certain pockets of the country (thanks to passionate parents), police are trained foremost to protect the safety of the community. When they observe someone behaving erratically who is a potential danger to themselves or a threat to others, they must treat the situation as though the individual is drunk, high, mentally ill, or all of the above—discerning autism is not a first response.

If you have concerns about your child being misperceived by law enforcement, make an appointment to meet with your local chief of police, or someone he or she designates, to discuss ways to keep your child safe in the community, and to explain your child's behaviors in a way that will demystify autism. Partner with your child in advance to discuss what you wish to share with the police and why. It is a preventive—not punitive or intimidating—measure. Look up the location of the police station on the Internet and invite your child to accompany you if you think it would be beneficial to do so. Many families have strong working relationships with local law enforcement and, in some cases, this kind of familiarity has averted serious consequences.

What do I do if he does get in trouble with the law?

Be certain you have educated your child about law enforcement officers, their role and responsibility, their desire to be friendly and helpful, and what to do when stopped by a police officer. Remember, if your child doesn't speak or communicate clearly, won't make eye contact, engages in repetitive actions, ambulates in an uncommon manner and runs away, or otherwise resists arrest, the encountering police officer will likely interpret the situation very differently than what your child intends—and may apply force to contain your child or fluster your child into confessing to something he didn't do. This kind of experience can be terrifying for a child with autism.

Be certain your child carries a photo ID and emergency contact information with him wherever he goes. If he is approached by a police officer, he should understand that he is not to run but should respond to the officer's desire to help by cooperating; the focus for both the officer and your child should be to reunite your child with you as efficiently as possible. One helpful website, Avoiding Unfortunate Situations, may be found online at http://policean-dautism.cjb.net/. It is hosted by Dennis Debbaudt, a former police officer, and offers a variety of educational resources for families of individuals with autism.

How do I help my child understand the sexual feelings he is having?

It is a positive thing that your child is discovering his sexuality—we are all sexual beings, even children. It is normal and natural for your child to wish to express his burgeoning sexuality, and the topic of masturbation was discussed in the chapter on physical well-being (Chapter 5). Still, your child's feelings of sexuality may be confusing. You will want to have a "birds and bees" dialogue with your child but also reinforce it with visuals—but not birds and bees literally! For the very young child, analogies with any previous experiences with kittens, puppies, or other animals delivering litters may be a place to start. For the preteen or adolescent, straight talk with plain and appropriate language, augmented with appropriate visuals, is best.

Sexual thoughts and feelings are private, and should only be shared with the consent of a close confidant(e). Your library or local video store may loan, at no cost, sexual education videos that you may screen and use to potentially supplement your conversation. Your personal or religious convictions will determine how you expect your child to express his or her sexuality. It is of utmost importance, though, that such discussions are comfortable for your child. Some adults with autism experience terribly frustrating, bizarre, or harmful thoughts about sexuality because they have been taught that it is "bad," "dirty," and hurtful.

My son is getting more and more interested in girls—how do I teach him to use self-control and to be respectful of others boundaries?

You would teach your child with autism about self-control and respectful boundaries the same as you would any of your children, except you should reinforce what you are verbally communicating with visuals and role-playing. A good start for young children is the approach of distinguishing a "good touch" from a "bad (or inappropriate) touch" of one's body parts by another person. However, caregivers, parents, and professionals often send very mixed messages to children with disabilities about appropriate touch because such children are often perceived as especially childlike, vulnerable, or cute. It is commonplace for young children with autism to be embraced or pulled into people's laps, sometimes by educators, classroom aides, and child care professionals. It's no wonder that a preteen accustomed to these kinds of confusing signals will find himself socially awkward for reciprocating what's been taught as acceptable. And when the child has fully grown and is no longer cute, people get up in arms when the same child grabs someone's breast when, in fact, we have encouraged this no-boundaries intimacy from the start. Make sure that you and all the adults in your child's life are aware of this possibility and do their best to help instill a proper sense of boundaries and respect in your child.

Can someone be autistic and gay? My teenage son doesn't seem interested in females but will comment on attractive male TV stars.

The answer to this question is the same as asking if someone who is born blind can also be gay. Or born with cerebral palsy. Or with blue eyes or olive skin. The answer is yes. Human sexuality is a grayscale as broad and diverse as that of the autism spectrum, and virtually anybody can be gay. Your child's budding homosexuality requires your compassionate sensitivity to support him to tame and refine his public reactions, and educate him about personal disclosure in the same ways you did about disclosing his autism diagnosis—both are natural human experiences.

Will my daughter with autism be able to conceive children as an adult woman, especially given the medications she takes?

If your daughter is healthy, menstruates as she should, and her female reproductive organs are free from anomalies, there is no reason why she wouldn't be able to conceive children as an adult woman. However, all medications come with risks and side effects of which you and your daughter should be keenly aware. If she is diagnosed with autism and a mental health issue such as bipolar disorder or even obsessive-compulsive disorder and she's taking an atypical antipsychotic medication, it could cause complications in her pregnancy. These medications could include Risperdal, Zyprexa, Seroquel, Geodon, Abilify, and Clozaril.

As always, consult with your doctor and thoroughly explore the interactions of the medications your daughter consumes. Nonmedicinal, holistic alternatives may be available as options if and when the time comes. Women with disabilities have a long history of being surgically sterilized without their consent to avert unwanted pregnancies in institutional congregate settings. Sterilization is an invasive, irrevocable, permanent procedure, and neuro-typical teenagers who are not prepared for the responsibilities of parenthood procreate every day, so sterilization should only be considered an option of last resort by today's standard's in lieu of the availability of contraceptives and proper education of such.

With the struggles my child is having in elementary school, is there hope for him in junior high, high school, and, one day, college?

Your fears for the future of your child's educational career likely lie more with the way he is being educated and perceived by his peers and teachers, and perhaps less about his abilities. If your child is just now in elementary school, channel your efforts into impressing on those with whom he spends most of his school day the three fundamental tenets of this book: presume intellect, practice prevention instead of intervention, and foster self-advocacy. Be certain to emphasize compassionate accommodations for sensory sensitivities, valuing passions, and identifying allies, all of which you have learned about in this book. It may not be at all easy to do, but your child is depending on you to advocate these principles on his behalf during his most formative years in order to poise him for future school success.

How do I help my child plan for college?

Higher education represents a huge time of transition for your child with autism. Even if your child's school years haven't been the best, it at least provided some measure of reliable structure and consistency. Depending on the extent to which your child is aware of college, the transition may be especially daunting if she believes that it is an all-or-nothing prospect; that is, college = leaving home. Quell your child's anxieties by discussing the myriad options for college such as online courses, commuting, beginning with one or two classes at the local community college, or correspondence courses. Trade and technical schools may also be options.

You will have, long before now, identified, nurtured, and cultivated your child's most passionate of interests. This action will now aid you in determining her most viable prospects for higher education and future employment. Partner with the school guidance counselor to consider those colleges that have strong programs that highlight curricula that build on your child's passions. You and your child may begin to gather visual information and logistical details about these schools over the Internet or by requesting hardcopy literature. Encourage your child to develop an itemized list of questions about her needs and concerns so that nothing is spontaneously overlooked when interviewing college personnel. Inquire about on-campus supports such as student advisors or counselors.

Campus visitations should be recorded by your child with photographs and videos, and the pros and cons should be discussed afterward with your child in the safety and comfort of your own home. You should also know that colleges are legally required to ensure equal opportunity for academically qualified students. Acceptable accommodations are other persons serving as note-takers or recording lectures, extra time for test-taking in distraction-free settings, and single dorm rooms for students for whom normal noise or the flicker of a fluorescent light amounts to sensory overload. *Realizing the College Dream with Autism or Asperger Syndrome: A Parent's Guide to Student Success* by Ann Palmer is one resource that may be helpful to you and your child.

What particular colleges are best at serving my child's needs?

It has become part of the culture of autism stereotypes to suggest that the local community college is the child with autism's only higher education option. And while colleges and universities should be progressive seats of higher learning, some are more progressive than others in providing individuals with invisible disabilities, not just physical disabilities, with social skills support. This support includes assistance in navigating college life, academically and socially. Those colleges that are gearing up to support the growing influx of newly enrolled students on the autism spectrum with innovative resource programs include:

- Youngstown State University (Ohio);
- Community College of Baltimore, Essex Campus (Maryland);
- Keene State College (New Hampshire);
- Marshall University (West Virginia);
- University of Minnesota;
- Boston University (Massachusetts);
- Carnegie Mellon (Pennsylvania);
- University of Pittsburgh (Pennsylvania); and
- George Mason at Arlington (Virginia).

How do I deal with feeling scared that my child will be exposed to drugs on campus?

This is an instance in which prevention instead of intervention should be part and parcel of your parenting repertoire. As you would with any of your children, and presuming the intellect of your child with autism, begin discussions about the dangers of drugs and alcohol at an early age. Show your child pictures of these substances and draw or show videos of situations in which they may potentially be offered. Reinforce that consuming these substances is not only illegal but will cause one to not be in control. Discuss and illustrate examples of the side effects of such drugs.

Some teens and adults with autism placate their mental health issues—feelings of worthlessness and depression—with nicotine, alcohol, and drugs to deaden the pain. It is important that you instill in your child self-knowledge of how best to cope with such challenges holistically and by relying on strong allies, in addition to knowing clearly how to communicate abject refusal if offered drugs on campus.

Will my child be able to have a job?

It is estimated that within the next decade 4 million people with autism will enter the workforce. With the advent of the Americans with Disabilities Act, employers are aware of making accommodations for people with physical disabilities because that's tangible and measurable. We are nowhere near making similar advances in accommodating people with neurological differences such as autism; so, the answer to this question depends on how the word "job" is defined. Employment for persons with autism may become more and more virtual and consist of using computers from home. The best case scenario is getting a job that taps into the expertise of one's most passionate interests. Regardless, there's no reason to believe that persons with autism shouldn't be gainfully employed—it's just that they'll have some pretty stiff competition. In what industry should they be most employable if they so choose? Foremost, the one into which they were born: autism.

There are those in the curious business of autism who are considered experts, and while many of these individuals are well intended, they are not autistic. They cannot presume to speak with intimacy about the autistic experience. They can only present their objective perspective based on observation and interaction with individuals who *are* autistic. It is these people with autism who are the true experts. Where employment within the expansive autism industry is concerned, there should be unlimited possibilities for listening to the wisdom and expertise of those who live it, allowing them to self-determine how their lives will and should be led—and fairly compensating them for their wealth of invaluable knowledge. If your child is developing self-advocacy skills, he or she may well opt to pursue this path.

What can I do to help my child prepare for a job interview?

Practice, practice, practice. You will not only need to coach your child about proper hygiene and attire in order to make a professional impression, but you will also have to address the social nuances of making eye contact, firmly shaking hands, and not monopolizing the conversation with superfluous information. Remember the waitress analogy for understanding verbal social interactions? It is like ordering from a menu: you don't tell the waitress your life story, you just give her enough information to get you what you want. This should also be the rule of thumb when your child is being interviewed—allow the interviewer to guide the direction of the conversation.

A thorough resume that itemizes your child's gifts and talents with tangible examples, supplemented by glowing endorsements of praise from former educators and staff, could augment discussion or be a starting point for conversation. Rehearse and role-play various scenarios with your child, and even use videotaping as an instructional strategy to improve how your child presents himself. *The Everything Parent's Guide to Children with Asperger's Syndrome* contains an in-depth chapter that explores these areas and others related to employment for people on the autism spectrum.

Is my child obligated to disclose her autism to prospective employers?

As previously noted, disclosure of one's autism diagnosis is a personal decision. There is no reason your child needs to tell her employer that she is autistic unless she—or you, both in agreement—feel it is necessary in order to underscore the rationale for specific workplace accommodations. Otherwise, it is nobody's business.

What can I do for my child who is despondent about always being passed over by employers?

The harsh reality of the big world is that first impressions and physical appearance do make a difference. But, above all else, people worship talent. Consider the unusual, eccentric, or even outrageous behavior with which some Hollywood and sports celebrities conduct themselves! Yet, oftentimes, all is overlooked, forgiven, or forgotten because of their appearance and enormously gifted propensity for what it is that they do so well.

When your child is being passed over by employers, are they employers that have an association with his area of passionate expertise, or some affiliation with your child's gifts and talents? It cannot be stressed enough to start cultivating your child with autism's gifts, talents, and areas of passion at as young an age as possible. In the case of the despondent child, begin exploring virtual employment opportunities on the Internet, self-employment, or consider employment opportunities that are self-contained and require little supervision or interaction with coworkers. Highlight your child's dependability, creative thinking ability, unique problem solving, strong work ethic, desire to please, and punctuality—all attractive attributes to any would-be employer.

I know my child is smart, so why is he only being hired as a janitor at a fast-food restaurant?

Your child is only being hired as a janitor at a fast-food restaurant because of myths and stereotypes about people with disabilities and their capabilities. Your child needs to shatter such antiquated mindsets by advocating the best application of what he has to offer the world through a paid position that matches his capabilities. If your child is not yet able to do so, he will require that you do so on his behalf. Remember, the big world is not waiting to accommodate your child's special needs; you've got to encourage your child to speak up for himself by respectfully but persistently requesting that compassionate accommodations be made.

Refuse to accept anything less than employment in which your child can sustain if not excel. If necessary, formally schedule a gathering of family and friends to assess your child's strengths, and develop an inventory of your child's gifts and talents. Your child's school guidance counselor should already be doing something similar. Your state's department of supported employment may be able to collaborate with you, but oftentimes such government offices are only knowledgeable about physical disabilities and are in dire need of autism-specific education and sensitivity. Some books that may be resources to you and your child include *Guide to Successful Employment for Individuals with Autism*, *Supported Employment Workbook: Using Individual Profiling and Job Matching*, and *Job-Hunting for the So-Called Handicapped or People Who Have Disabilities*.

My child has autism and a mental health diagnosis— how can I help her deal with both in adulthood?

You can support your adult child with autism and a mental health diagnosis by being among your child's most ardent of allies. It is commonplace for adults on the autism spectrum to grapple with the kinds of psychological issues detailed in this book's mental health chapter (Chapter 6). Unchecked and untreated, it can lead to depression, self-deprecating thoughts, and suicidal tendencies. In addition to your support, ensure that your child is fully and exhaustively well informed about her diagnoses and medications she may consume (and their side effects), and that she follows a plan of holistic wellness that includes proper diet, rest, and exercise. Your child should be well versed enough to recognize her own manifesting mental health symptoms to distinguish them clearly from symptoms of her autism. As mentioned previously, you cannot insulate your child from harm around the clock, but you can make certain that your child knows she is unconditionally loved, admired, and respected, and that she has you and others to call on if she ever feels stuck.

Will my child grow out of his autism by adulthood?

As some people with autism age, they become more adept at taming and refining their autistic symptoms in order to blend, assimilate, and pass for "normal." Your child may or may not have this as an endeavor of any priority. If your child's autistic symptoms become less noticeable as he grows and matures, so be it; but please know that no one "grows out of" autism anymore than they grow out of their skin color. It is a natural, lifelong experience and, as a parent, you would do well not to peg your hopes and expectations on anything other than this.

I have heard several news stories about parents murdering their kids with autism—why is this happening?

It has been speculated that the recent spate of parents who have murdered their children with autism (and in a couple of instances,

taken their own lives as well) have succumbed to the pressures of an
unyielding society that values perfection and normalcy. It is a powerful
and seductive lure when parents of children with autism are promised
"recovery" for their children; but examples of kids with autism
completely fading their so-called autistic traits are rare. Can you
imagine the tremendous guilt imposed on the parent whose child with
autism is *not* making significant advances while enrolled in programming that proffers a "cure"? Many parents belabor what they could or
should be doing differently to support their child. Know your child
best, trust your parental intuitions, rely on your gut feelings, and
follow your heart in discerning what is right and true and good and
kind. Murder and suicide are not options; the world *needs* people like
your child in it—magnificent, gorgeous human beings who can teach
us tolerance, patience, compassion, and acceptance of diversity.

What is *person-centered planning* and how can it benefit my child?

Person-centered planning (PCP) is a process that can support your
child with autism in her transition to adulthood, higher education,
or the workforce. PCP provides a blueprint for mapping your child's
next steps by focusing on the positives, crafted by those persons who
know your child best and directed by your child's wants, needs, and
desires. The PCP process is not conducted by a counselor or professional (unless you so desire) but, instead, by you, your child and
those who know her best. The outcome of the PCP is aimed at
helping your child attain a desirable future and pressing to advocate
for ingenuity, creativity, and the change of established systems in
order to gratify that future. That vision must be the individual's—not
what others want or believe for her.

PCP is an open-ended process that occurs when committed and
caring people come together to brainstorm solutions, devoid of

roadblock statements like "We can't because...." An actual document should be drafted that assigns roles, responsibilities, and time frames for initiating, implementing, and exploring the steps necessary to begin realizing the individual's goals for the future. There are many names and formats by which PCP is referred. Training Resource Network, Inc. (www.trninc.com or 1-866-823-9800) is but one resource that offers PCP materials to inspire individuals and their support teams in the planning process.

Can I appoint someone to be my child's legal guardian?

In planning for their child's future, many parents of those with autism find peace of mind while they are living in knowing that a guardian has been assigned to monitor the well-being of their son or daughter, particularly if something unexpected should happen to either parent. Guardianship may be defined as the legal relationship between a competent adult and a person over the age of eighteen who is unable to make decisions for himself or reliably give consent; your child's autism could qualify him for guardianship. Rights to make such decisions on behalf of the person with autism (or other qualifying disability) are court appointed in varying capacities and degrees of responsibility. Depending on how guardianship is defined in your home state, the types of responsibility may be categorized as a guardian of a person, full guardianship, limited guardianship, and temporary guardianship. All forms of guardianship are intended to protect and uphold the rights and best interests of the person for whom guardianship is deemed appropriate.

To initiate the guardianship process, a petition of guardianship should be completed and filed with the county court in the jurisdiction within which the individual resides (or the individual's parents if the person lives away from home). A guardian may include (in order of preference):

- an individual or organization approved by the person requiring guardianship,
- your spouse,
- your adult child,
- another parent as provided by your will,
- a family relative with whom your child has lived for at least six months prior to filing the petition for guardianship,
- someone nominated by your child's caregiver, or
- a state government agency.

A guardian should be prepared to be actively involved in the life of the individual to whom they have been appointed; in other words, be certain you are appointing someone who understands autism and your child's unique way of being. Guardianship is terminated by the court only, but the petition to do so may be advanced by anyone, including the person with autism. One website that may prove useful in pursuing the issue of guardianship is that of the National Guardianship Association at www.guardianship.org.

What will become of my child after I die?

All parents wonder about the future of their children—will they be loved, have a job, have children? But as the parent of a child with autism in particular, you may find yourself agonizing over your inability to predict your child's future life. But then, no one can guarantee predictable outcomes for their children's future, whether they have autism or not. Legally, arrange for provisions of your child's financial future in your will, establish a trust, appoint a trustee, and explore your child's eligibility for Medicaid, Supplemental Security Income (SSI), and Social Security Disability Insurance (SSDI) if you haven't already. Some of the organizations listed as resources at the back of this book provide contacts or literature that can aid in estate planning for your child.

Making philosophical peace with the reality of your child's future after you're gone may be aided by adhering to the following:

- learning all you can about autism,
- joining an autism support group,
- taking one day at a time,
- focusing on now, being in the moment with your child,
- celebrating successes,
- being open to disappointment but not failure,
- cultivating strong allies for your child (not necessarily siblings),
- having faith in your child, and
- surrendering to the fact that some things are beyond your control.

Trust that your child with autism will make his own way, in his own time. He will touch and inspire many during his life's journey. He will defrost unkind hearts, bridge gaps in communication, and give cause to celebrate the humanity in us all. And know, above all else, that his unique and different way of being will not be without purpose in this world.

WRITTEN SOCIAL NARRATIVES

Throughout *The Autism Answer Book,* reference has been made to ensuring that you are reinforcing what you communicate verbally to your child with autism in ways that he best thinks, learns, and processes information. Oftentimes, this means using pictures, words, or pictures paired with words, among other techniques. If your child is an auditory learner instead, tape record these and similar stories for listening replay. What follows in this appendix are some sample stories that may address some issues and concerns not covered in the text of this book. You, your child, and his team of supporters will be obliged to write additional stories to address issues as they arise. The concept of written social narratives, or social stories, was developed by Carol Gray, a special educator, author, and trainer. Ms. Gray's website and books are listed in the appendixes that follow.

The written social narratives in this section may be copied and used to demystify certain aspects of daily life for your child. You may adapt them to suit your needs; for example, if a story is too long, shorten it or reprint it with a sentence at a time on a page, or have your child personally invest in it by illustrating or videotaping reenactments of it. The three themes of this book are reflected in the outcomes of these stories. Presuming intellect, you should read each story with your child, allowing him to follow the words or even read it to you if he can. Phase out the use of each story as your child demonstrates his understanding until the story is no longer necessary. In keeping with prevention instead of intervention, review the needed story *prior to* entering into a situation in which it is required most. The final outcome will result in a fostering of self-advocacy as your child masters control over anxieties, fears, and concerns that may conspire to hinder him socially.

It's Important to Poop

Every living creature has bowel movements, or poops.

This means that all animals, birds, insects, and fish poop. I can name some favorite animals when I think about this.

This means all people poop too. Every single person I know poops. It is natural and normal to poop every day.

When I poop, my body is getting rid of what it doesn't need, like when I throw out garbage after I eat lunch in school.

My body makes poop after it takes out all the vitamins and other good things it needs from the food I eat. What's left over is garbage or waste.

If I try to hold in my poop, I could make my body very sick. My stomach may hurt, or I may not be able to eat very well.

When I feel like I might need to poop, I will try to get to the bathroom right away. I will try to poop in the toilet because everyone does this.

Pooping every day is good. It is okay and will keep my body healthy.

© 2007 William Stillman, The Autism Answer Book

Clean Hands

It is important for me to have clean hands.

When I lick my fingers and touch things, my hands are not clean.

When I put my hands down my pants, my hands are not clean.

Hands that are not clean carry bad germs that can make people sick.

I must wash my hands if I lick my fingers and touch things, or if I put my hands down my pants.

When I wash my hands, it will help to get rid of the bad germs.

When I wash my hands, I may not get sick or make others sick.

It is okay to lick my fingers when I am alone in my room.

It is okay to put my hands in my pants when I am alone in my room.

I just need to remember to wash my hands afterward.

It is bad manners to lick my fingers and touch things or put my hands in my pants when other people can see me.

I want people to know that I am smart.

I want people to know that I have good manners.

I Miss [Whoever has Passed Away]

I miss _____ very much.

He/She died on [fill in complete date] .

Now he/she is in Heaven.

In Heaven everyone is happy, and full of love and joy.

In Heaven, no one is angry or unhappy.

Even though I know _____ is happy in Heaven, I still miss him/her.

This is okay.

When I miss _____, I can:

- Cry if I feel like it.
- Look at his/her picture and remember happy times with him/her, like _____.
- Talk to him/her in Heaven, and tell him/her I miss him/her and still love him/her.
- Talk to mom/dad/caregiver about my feelings, and they will listen.

Everyone I know has someone who died that they miss very much.

It is okay to cry and miss and talk about people/pets who died that we love.

Masturbation

My body is my own.

My body is beautiful.

My body is made up of many different parts, inside and out.

Inside parts are like my heart and stomach.

Outside parts are like my arms and legs.

The outside parts that are between my legs and covered by my underwear are called my sexual organs.

My sexual organs are my penis and my testicles.

Many boys and men touch, rub, or gently pull their penis. When this happens, their penis usually gets bigger and harder. The same thing may happen to me. This is normal and okay.

If I touch, rub, or gently pull my penis, this is called masturbation. Many boys and men masturbate. Masturbation is a choice that is my own to make.

If I choose to masturbate it may be because I am thinking about sex.

It may be because I am thinking about another person.

It may be because I want to feel good.

It may be because I want some time alone with my body.

It may be for other reasons.

When I masturbate, I may feel excited inside. I may breathe harder. I may breathe faster. This is normal and okay.

When I masturbate, I may get so excited that my penis ejaculates. This means that something white and wet comes out of the opening in the tip of my penis. It is called semen or sperm. I may not ejaculate semen or sperm every time I masturbate. But if I do, this is normal and okay.

If I choose to masturbate, I will try to remember to masturbate in a private place. This means I will go to a place where there are no other people around. This means I will go to a place where I can be alone with my body. A private place may be my bedroom or a bathroom.

People masturbate in a private place because sexual organs are private. People wear underwear and clothes to keep their sexual organs private. People expect one another to masturbate in a private place. People will also expect me to masturbate in a private place. It is like a rule.

A place that is not private is a place with other people around me. If I touch my sexual organs when I'm in a place that is not private—even if I'm wearing pants—people may be upset. They may laugh at me. They may be angry. They may report me to the police. They may not think I am smart.

They may think these things because people expect one another to masturbate in a private place. If I masturbate in a place that is not private, I am breaking a rule that people expect me to know.

I will try not to touch my sexual organs, or put my hands in my pants, or masturbate in a place that is not private. I will try to remember to masturbate only in a private place. Masturbation is a choice that is my own to make. It is normal and okay.

© 2007 William Stillman, The Autism Answer Book

Reporting Pain

My body is my own. My body is beautiful. I will try to take good care of my body so I can enjoy good health all my life.

My body is made up of many different parts inside and out.

Inside parts are like my heart and stomach.

Outside parts are like my arms and legs.

Sometimes my body is hurt. When my body is hurt, I may be in pain or I may feel discomfort, like an ache or a pinching feeling.

The part of my body that hurts could be an inside or an outside part.

I know when my body is hurt because my body will give me a signal.

A signal is a sign that something is wrong with a part of my body or that a part of my body is hurt.

This is normal.

Another word for signal is symptom.

Everybody's body gives them symptoms or signals when a part of their body is hurt or when they are feeling pain or discomfort.

If I don't report the pain, it could get worse.

If I don't report the pain, it is difficult for others to help me feel better.

A symptom or signal that my stomach is hurting may be that I am unable to eat or I feel a burning in my stomach or I throw up.

A symptom or signal for my throat hurting may be scratchiness or burning and difficulty swallowing or eating.

A symptom or signal that my head is hurting may be pain in my forehead.

A symptom or signal that my acid reflex is causing me pain or discomfort may be when I have burning in both my throat and stomach.

It is important for me to report when my body gives me signals that it hurts or is in pain.

I can report when my body is giving me a signal and I am in pain or have discomfort.

One way I can report this pain or discomfort by pointing to a picture of my body that is hurting me. Another way is to point to the place on my own body where I feel pain or discomfort. Another way is to write on paper where I am feeling pain or discomfort.

When I report this pain, others will know how to help me get relief from the pain. This may be by getting extra rest. It may be by taking a warm bath or shower. It may be by taking medicine to make the pain go away. It may be other ways too.

Sometimes, I might have to go to the doctor so he can give me a different kind of medicine to help the pain go away. The doctor will know best of all how to help me feel better.

Sensory Overload

Every day I hear and see and feel many, many things.

Some things are good and make me feel happy.

Other things, like loud noises or being touched, may make me feel bad.

I may feel like screaming or doing something I know I shouldn't do.

When I feel bad because of too much noise or too many people touching me, I will try to tell someone about it.

That is better than screaming or doing something I shouldn't do.

When I feel like I'm getting upset because of noise or people or other things like that, I will try to remember to tell someone.

That way, I can feel better and they will understand me.

© *2007 William Stillman, The Autism Answer Book*

Respect

All people deserve respect.

Respect is when people treat one another with kindness.

Disrespect is when people do things like angry swearing, hitting, pinching, spitting, or biting one another. Disrespect makes people feel really bad.

Respect works in two ways.

The first way is: people can respect me.

The second way is: I can respect other people.

When people understand me, they respect me.

When people treat me like another good human being, they respect me.

When people like me just the way I am, they respect me.

I can respect other people.

I can try to remember that each person has his or her own thoughts.

I can try to remember that all people deserve respect.

I can try to remember that no one wants disrespect.

I show respect when I try to be polite and kind. I show respect when I try not to swear or say bad things. I show respect when I do not hit, kick, bite, pinch, or break things.

All people deserve respect.

Sleeping in My Own Bed

When my family goes to sleep at night, my Mommy and Daddy sleep in their own bed and I sleep in mine.

Sometimes when I wake up during the night, I get in bed with Mommy and Daddy.

I like to do this, but when I do this it wakes up Mommy and Daddy.

It may make it hard for them to sleep again.

When people don't get enough sleep, they may feel very tired, sick, or grouchy.

It is important for me to try to sleep in my own bed all night long. If I wake up during the night, instead of getting in bed with Mommy and Daddy, I can:

- Get a drink of water from the bathroom.
- Go to the bathroom.
- Lay in bed and pray.
- Lay in bed and think about my favorite movies/cartoons/video games.

Starting [day/month/year], I will try to stay in my own bed all night long so Mommy and Daddy can sleep in their own bed.

Trespassing

My home and yard is my property, and no one else's.

It is the same for other people, like our neighbors.

Their home and yard is their property and no one else's.

Mom/dad/caregiver will show me where my yard begins and ends.

If it will help me remember, together we can mark where my yard begins and ends.

If I leave my yard and walk onto someone else's property without those people saying it is okay, it is called TRESPASSING.

Most people already understand the rules about not trespassing on other people's property.

If I trespass without the other people saying it is okay, it can be very upsetting for the people who live there. They may be angry that I am in their yard. They may think I'm a burglar. They may think I'm dangerous. They may call the police. They may think I'm not smart. They may think I don't know the rules about trespassing.

I might be very upset if a stranger trespassed on my property. I will try to remember not to trespass on other people's property. I will try to remember to stay in my own yard.

© 2007 William Stillman, The Autism Answer Book

Turning Off Lights

Everyday my mom/dad/caregiver turns on lights at home.

When they turn on lights, it is to help them see clearly in the dark.

The light helps them to see what they are doing, like reading or writing.

When I walk by and turn off the light, they can no longer see what they are doing.

This may make them angry or upset because I have stopped them from seeing clearly.

They have to get up and turn the light back on.

When I turn off lights, they may think I am being bad, or that I am not as smart as I am.

I will try to show respect by not turning off lights when others are using them.

Wearing My Pants

When I go outside of my home, or have visitors in my home, I put pants on.

People wear pants to protect their skin, to keep warm, and to keep their sexual organs private.

People expect one another to wear pants outside of their homes, of when they have visitors. It is like a rule.

If I do not wear my pants, people may be upset. They may laugh at me. They may be angry. They may report me to the police. They may not think I am smart.

They may think these things because people expect one another to wear pants.

If I do not wear pants in front of other people, I am breaking a rule that people expect me to know.

I will try to remember to wear my pants outside of my home or when I have visitors.

When People Leave

There are people in my life who come and go.

Sometimes I wish some people would stay longer.

When people leave me, it may be because:

- They got a new job.
- They moved away.
- They don't have as much time to spend with me as they used to.
- It may be for other reasons.

This happens to everyone.

When people leave me, it is not my fault.

When some people leave me, I may miss them and feel unhappy.

It natural to feel unhappy, and that is okay.

When people leave me, I will try to remember that they have reasons.

When people leave me, I will try to remember that I am a good person, and it is not my fault.

© *2007 William Stillman, The Autism Answer Book*

Everyone Makes Mistakes

Most everyone tries to do their best.

Even though I try to do my best, I may make mistakes.

Everyone makes mistakes.

Making mistakes is okay.

Mistakes can be fixed by me or with help.

People make mistakes every single day.

My mom, dad, grandma, and brothers make mistakes.

My teachers and helpers make mistakes.

Other kids I know make mistakes.

All of these people make mistakes because no one is perfect.

I don't have to upset myself trying to be perfect because I am human.

I will try not to take up time worrying about always doing perfect work.

I will just try to do my best.

© *2007 William Stillman, The Autism Answer Book*

Eating at School

When I am in school, I eat breakfast and lunch there.

When I eat in school, an adult is with me.

I do not need permission to eat every bite.

When I eat in school, I will try to eat on my own.

I don't need to permission to eat every bite at home.

When I eat in school, I will try to eat on my own, like at home.

I can eat as much or as little as I want in school.

But I don't need permission to eat every bite.

I can do this on my own.

© 2007 William Stillman, The Autism Answer Book

There's a Lot I Can Do

I can do a lot of good things.

Some of the things I can do include _____.

When I do good things, I feel good about myself.

Sometimes, I may feel like I don't want to try to do something.

When this happens, I may feel anxious or upset, or like I can't do it.

Instead of feeling this way, I will try something new.

I will think to myself, "I can do a lot of good things."

I will think to myself, "I will try."

If I try something and mess up, that is okay.

No one does everything they try perfectly.

If I try something and need help, I can ask mom/dad/caregiver for help.

When I do good things, I feel good about myself for trying.

© 2007 William Stillman, The Autism Answer Book

Transitioning to Living in the Community

Many people move out of their mother and father's house when they grow up.

I am grown up too and have a house of my very own.

I can still call my family on the phone whenever I want.

I can still visit my family too.

They can visit me in my new house.

The address of my new home is _____.

This house is my house, and does not belong to anyone else.

It does not belong to my staff.

It does not belong to my parents.

It is my house for as long as I want to live there.

No one can take my house away from me.

Having my own house means I must take care of it.

I will try to keep every room of my house nice and clean.

I will try to take care of my yard by mowing it.

I will try to respect my house by not throwing things or breaking things.

I may have other ideas about how I can care for my house.

These ideas may be chores, like vacuuming or grocery shopping.

These ideas may be buying new things for my house and my yard.

These ideas may be changing things inside my house to make it the way I want it.

I can share my ideas with my staff.

My staff may also have ideas for me to think about too, but I don't have to say yes to their ideas if I don't want to.

© *2007 William Stillman, The Autism Answer Book*

Appendix B INTERNET RESOURCES

The following list of organization and specialist websites is but a sampling of the wide variety of Internet resources pertaining to the autism spectrum.

Asperger Syndrome Education Network, Inc., headquartered in New Jersey. *www.aspennj.org*

Asperger's Association of New England. Fosters awareness, respect, acceptance, and support for people with Asperger's and their families. *www.aane.org*

Autism Living and Working. Pennsylvania-based group of parents and others who support community living and housing for people with autism. *www.autismlivingworking.org*

Autism National Committee. *www.autcom.org*

Autism Network International. A self-help and advocacy organization run by people with autism for people on the autism spectrum. *www.ani.ac*

Autism One Radio. Online radio programming established by parents. *www.autismone.org/radio*

The Autism Perspective (TAP). Website for the magazine *The Autism Perspective*. *www.theautismperspective.org*

The Autism Service Center. A national autism hotline and website. *www.autismservicescenter.org*

Autism Society of America. *www.autism-society.org*

Autism Spectrum Quarterly. Autism "magajournal" with articles by, for, and about individuals with autism. *www.ASQuarterly.com*

Autism Talk. An online community with a variety of discussion categories on all aspects of autism. *www.autismtalk.net*

Autism Today. Latest news and resources for autism and autism-related issues. *www.autismtoday.com*

Autism/Asperger's Digest Magazine. *www.autismdigest.com*

Autistics.Org. Resources by and for persons on the autism spectrum, including many links to other self-advocates' websites. *www.autistics.org*

Breaking the Barriers. A website supported by TASH (an international organization for persons with disabilities and their supporters) that includes vision statements, a call to action, and personal stories. *www.breaking-the-barriers.org*

The Bubel/Aiken Foundation. *www.thebubelaikenfoundation.org*

Chat Autism. A chat and community forum for those with autism and their families. *www.chatautism.com*

Cure Autism Now. *www.cureautismnow.org*

The Dan Marino Foundation. *www.danmarinofoundation.org*

Donna Williams. A prominent autism self-advocate and author. *www.donnawilliams.net*

The Doug Flutie Jr. Foundation for Autism, Inc. *www.dougflutiejrfoundation.org*

Facilitated Communication Institute, Syracuse University, New York, Dr. Douglas Biklen, Director. *http://soeweb.syr.edu/thefci*

Families for Early Autism Treatment. *www.feat.org*

The Global and Regional Asperger Syndrome Partnership (GRASP). An informational, educational, and advocacy organization operated by persons on the autism spectrum. *www.grasp.org*

The Gray Center. Website of special educator and social stories founder Carol Gray. *www.thegraycenter.org*

Lianne Holliday Willey. Asperger's syndrome self-advocate and author. *www.aspie.com*

Looking Up. Monthly international autism newsletter. *www.lookingupautism.org*

MAAP Services. Covers autism, Asperger's syndrome, and pervasive developmental disorder. *www.maapservices.org*

National Alliance for Autism Research. *www.naar.org*

National Association of Councils on Developmental Disabilities. *www.nacdd.org*

National Institutes of Health autism site. *www.ninds.nih.gov/health_and_medical/disorders/autism.htm*

National Parent to Parent Network. *www.P2PUSA.org*

Networks for Training and Development. Pennsylvania-based training and resource organization for caregivers of people with differences, including autism, that supports the use of augmentative and alternative communication methods. *www.networksfortraining.org*

Neurodiversity.com. A demagogic collection of information "honoring the variety of human wiring" that also includes national news reports on the abuses committed against persons with autism. *www.neurodiversity.com*

Online Asperger's Syndrome Information and Support (OASIS). Website created by parents. *www.aspergersyndrome.org*

Ontario Adult Autism Research and Support Network (OAARSN). *www.ont-autism.uoguelph.ca*

Police and Autism. A web page about autism and law enforcement. *http://policeandautism.cjb.net/avoiding.html*

Stephen Shore. Asperger's syndrome self-advocate, consultant, and author. *www.autismasperger.net*

Spectrum Publications. Home of *Spectrum* magazine. *www.spectrumpublications.com*

Temple Grandin. Perhaps the best known autism self-advocate and bestselling author. *www.templegrandin.com*

Tony Attwood. Acknowledged Asperger's syndrome authority. *www.tonyattwood.com*

Transition Map. A website by Pennsylvania professionals for educators supporting high school students with differences who are transitioning to adult life. *www.transitionmap.org*

Unlocking Autism. Website with a listserv to connect parents, teens, and adults with autism and Asperger's. *www.unlockingautism.org*

U.S. Department of Education. *www.ed.gov*

William Stillman. Website of Asperger's and autism self-advocate, author, consultant and presenter. *www.williamstillman.com*

Wright's Law. Website of Peter Wright, Esquire, an expert on special education. *www.wrightslaw.org*

Appendix C RECOMMENDED READING

Aston, Maxine. *Asperger's in Love: Couple Relationships and Family Affairs* (London: Jessica Kingsley Publishers, Ltd., 2003).

Attwood, Tony. *Asperger's Syndrome: A Guide for Parents and Professionals* (London: Jessica Kingsley Publishers, Ltd., 1998).

Berger, Dorita S. *Music Therapy, Sensory Integration and the Autistic Child* (London: Jessica Kingsley Publishers, Ltd., 2002).

Biklen, Douglas. *Autism and the Myth of the Person Alone* (New York: New York University Press, 2005).

Birch, Jen. *Congratulations! It's Asperger Syndrome* (London: Jessica Kingsley Publishers, Ltd., 2003).

Boyd, Brenda. *Parenting a Child with Asperger Syndrome: 200 Tips and Strategies* (London: Jessica Kingsley Publishers, Ltd., 2003).

Brunett, Rhonda. *From Autism to All-Star* (Carol Stream, IL: Specialty Publishing Company, 2004).

Cohen, Shirley. *Targeting Autism* (Berkeley: University of California Press, 1998).

Faherty, Catherine. *Asperger's: What Does It Mean to Me? Structured Teaching Ideas for Home and School* (Arlington, TX: Future Horizons, 2000).

Grandin, Temple. *Thinking in Pictures and Other Reports from My Life with Autism* (New York: Doubleday, 1995).

Gray, Carol. *The New Social Story Book: Illustrated Edition* (Arlington, TX: Future Horizons, 2000).

_____. *The Original Social Story Book* (Arlington, TX: Future Horizons, 1994).

Greenspan, Stanley I. *Engaging Autism: Helping Children Relate, Communicate and Think with the DIR Floortime Approach* (Cambridge, MA: Da Capo Lifelong Books, 2006).

Hamilton, Lynn M. *Facing Autism: Giving Parents Reasons for Hope and Guidance for Help* (Colorado Springs, CO: Waterbrook Press, 2000).

Hill, David A., and Martha R. Leary (Anne M. Donnellan, Series Editor). *Movement Disturbance: A Clue to Hidden Competencies in Persons Diagnosed with Autism and Other Developmental Disabilities* (Madison, WI: DRI Press, 1993).

Holliday Willey, Liane. *Asperger Syndrome in the Family* (London: Jessica Kingsley Publishers, Ltd., 2001).

_____. *Pretending to be Normal: Living with Asperger's Syndrome* (London: Jessica Kingsley Publishers, Ltd., 1999).

Jackson, Luke. *Freaks, Geeks and Asperger's Syndrome: A User's Guide to Adolescence* (London: Jessica Kingsley Publishers, Ltd., 2002).

Kephart, Beth. *A Slant of Sun: One Child's Courage* (New York: W. W. Norton & Company, 1998).

Kern Kogel, Lynn, and LaZebnik, Claire. *Overcoming Autism: Finding the Answers, Strategies, and Hope That Can Transform a Child's Life* (New York: Penguin Books, 2005).

Lawson, Wendy. *Build Your Own Life: A Self-Help Guide for Individuals with Asperger's Syndrome* (London: Jessica Kingsley Publishers, Ltd., 2003).

Meyer, Roger. *Asperger Syndrome Employment Workbook: An Employment Workbook for Adults with Asperger Syndrome* (London: Jessica Kingsley Publishers, Ltd., 2000).

Moor, Julia. *Playing, Laughing and Learning with Children on the Autism Spectrum: A Practical Resource of Play Ideas for Parents and Carers* (London: Jessica Kingsley Publishers, Ltd., 2002).

Moyes, Rebecca A. *Addressing the Challenging Behavior of Children with High-Functioning Autism/Asperger Syndrome in the Classroom: A Guide for Teachers and Parents* (London: Jessica Kingsley Publishers, Ltd., 2002).

——————. *Incorporating Social Skills in the Classroom: A Guide for Teachers and Parents of Children with High-Functioning Autism and Asperger's Syndrome* (London: Jessica Kingsley Publishers, Ltd., 2001).

Notbohm, Ellen. *Ten Things Every Child with Autism Wishes You Knew* (Arlington, TX: Future Horizons, 2005).

——————. *Ten Things Your Student with Autism Wishes You Knew* (Arlington, TX: Future Horizons, 2006).

O'Neill, Jasmine Lee. *Through the Eyes of Aliens: A Book about Autistic People* (London: Jessica Kingsley Publishers, Ltd., 1999).

Papolos, Demitri F., and Janice Papolos. *The Bipolar Child: The Definitive and Reassuring Guide to Childhood's Most Misunderstood Disorder* (New York: Broadway Books, 1999).

Pyles, Lise. *Hitchhiking through Asperger Syndrome: How to Help Your Child When No One Else Will* (London: Jessica Kingsley Publishers, Ltd., 2001).

Sabin, Ellen. *The Autism Acceptance Book: Being a Friend to Someone with Autism* (Watering Can, 2006).

Senator, Susan. *Making Peace with Autism: One Family's Story of Struggle, Discovery and Unexpected Gifts* (Trumpeter Books, 2006).

Shore, Stephen M. *Beyond the Wall: Personal Experiences with Autism and Asperger Syndrome* (Shawnee Mission, KS: Autism Asperger Publishing Company, 2003).

_____, and Rastelli, Linda G. *Understanding Autism for Dummies* (New York: Hungry Minds/Wiley, 2006).

Sicile-Kira, Chantal, and Grandin, Temple. *Autism Spectrum Disorders: The Complete Guide to Understanding Autism, Asperger's Syndrome, Pervasive Developmental Disorder, and Other ASDs* (Perigee Trade, 2004).

Stanford, Ashley. *Asperger Syndrome and Long-Term Relationships* (London: Jessica Kingsley Publishers, Ltd., 2002).

Stillman, William. *Demystifying the Autistic Experience: A Humanistic Introduction for Parents, Caregivers and Educators* (London: Jessica Kingsley Publishers, Ltd., 2002).

_____. *The Everything Parent's Guide to Children with Asperger's Syndrome: Help, Hope and Guidance* (Avon, MA: Adams Media, 2005).

_____. *The Everything Parent's Guide to Children with Bipolar Disorder: Professional, Reassuring Advice to Help You Understand and Cope* (Avon, MA: Adams Media, 2005).

Winter, Matt. *Asperger's Syndrome: What Teachers Need to Know* (London: Jessica Kingsley Publishers, Ltd., 2003).

Zysk, Veronica, and Notbohm, Ellen. *1001 Great Ideas for Teaching and Raising Children with Autism Spectrum Disorders* (Arlington, TX: Future Horizons, 2004).

Index

D

loss, 283, 290–91
masturbation, 284–85
mistakes, 291
pain, reporting, 285–86
pica behavior, 85
respect, 287–88
right and wrong, 190–91
self-affirmation, 292
sensory overload, 287
sleeping, 288
trespassing, 288–89
Social reciprocations, 203
Social Security Disability
  Insurance (SSDI), 278
Social skills training, 160–61
Social stories, 161–62
Sound sensitivities. *See* Hearing
  sensitivities
Spanking, 187
Special schools, 231
Special treatment, 187–88
Spectrum disorder, 6
Speech delay, 48, 50, 167
Speech problems
  encouragement and, 51–52
  assistance for, 50–51
  regression, 64
  repetitive questions, 59–60
  repetitive speech, 58–59
  speech delay, 48, 50, 167
  See also Communication;
    Verbal communication

Speech therapy
  communication, 48, 51, 59
  diagnosis and evaluation, 26
  treatment options, 154, 167,
    172
Spirituality, 35
Spouses
  behavior problems and, 113
  diagnosis and evaluation,
    44–45
  discipline and, 179–80, 182,
    183
Stereotypes, 12, 13, 14, 15,
  24–25, 40, 44, 80, 111, 177,
  181, 250, 251, 260, 262,
  269–270, 274
Sterilization, 267–68
Stigma, 44
Stimming, 59, 78–81
Strangers, 57–58, 139
Substance abuse, 270–71
Suicide, 276
Summer vacation, 256–57
Supervision, 21
Supplemental Security Income
  (SSI), 278
Supplements, 119–20
Support, 38–39
Support services, 168–69
Symptoms, 3–4, 24–25

T

About the Author

William Stillman is the author of Sourcebooks' *Autism and the God Connection: Redefining the Autistic Experience through Extraordinary Accounts of Spiritual Giftedness* (2006). His other books include *The Everything Parent's Guide to Children with Asperger's Syndrome: Help, Hope and Guidance* (2005), *The Everything Parent's Guide to Children with Bipolar Disorder: Professional, Reassuring Advice to Help You Understand and Cope* (2005), and *Demystifying the Autistic Experience: A Humanistic Introduction for Parents, Caregivers and Educators* (2002), which has been highly praised by the autism and self-advocacy communities. Stillman also writes a column, "Through the Looking Glass," for the national quarterly publication *The Autism Perspective*, and is on that magazine's advisory board.

As an adult with Asperger's syndrome, a mild "cousin" of autism, Stillman's message of reverence and respect has touched thousands nationally through his acclaimed autism workshops and private consultations.

Stillman has a BS in education from Millersville University in Pennsylvania, and has worked to support people with different ways of being since 1987. He was formerly the Pennsylvania Department of Public Welfare's Office of Mental Retardation's statewide point person for children with intellectual impairment, mental health issues, and autism.

Stillman is founder of the Pennsylvania Autism Self Advocacy Coalition (PASAC), which endeavors to educate and advise state and local government, law enforcement, educators, and the medical community about the autism spectrum from the "inside out." He served on Pennsylvania's Autism Task Force, and is on the advisory boards for Autism Living and Working, The Asperger's Syndrome Alliance of Pennsylvania, and the Youth Advocate Programs' National Autism Committee. He is the coordinator for a Pennsylvania-based meeting group of individuals who use augmentative and alternative communication. Stillman has also been a consultant to Temple University for the development of Youth Advocate Programs' Therapeutic Staff Support curriculum, which will set the standard by which mental health workers in Pennsylvania will be trained to support children and adolescents with autism and mental health issues.

In his work to support those who love and care for individuals with autism and Asperger's syndrome, Stillman sets a tone for our collective understanding of the autistic experience in ways that are unprecedented. Autism should not be defined as an affliction endured by sufferers, but as a truly unique and individual experience to be respected and appreciated by all. In so doing, Stillman highlights the exquisite sensitivities of our most valuable, wise and loving teachers.

William Stillman's website is www.williamstillman.com.